Indoor Air Quality and Human Health

Indoor Air Quality and Human Health

Isaac Turiel

Stanford University Press, Stanford, California

Stanford University Press
Stanford, California
© 1985 by the Board of Trustees of the
Leland Stanford Junior University
Printed in the United States of America
Original printing 1985
Last figure below indicates year of this printing:
95   94   93   92   91   90   89   88   87   86

CIP data appear at the end of the book

Preface

The primary impetus for writing this book came about as I discovered a lack of publicly available and understandable information on the subject of indoor air pollution and its public health effects. Through my work at Lawrence Berkeley Laboratory, I found that many people outside the research community were interested in learning of the results of the laboratory's research and wished to apply this knowledge to their own situations. My colleagues and I often received requests from architects, ventilation engineers, health professionals, reporters, and members of the general public for information on indoor air pollution.

My objectives are to provide general information on indoor air pollution sources and the pollutants commonly found indoors, and also to explore the potential health effects arising from exposure to these pollutants. At this time it is not possible to predict accurately the health risks for people living in homes with air quality problems relative to those living in homes without such problems. However, guidance can be given as to what exposure levels are likely to cause adverse health effects and what control techniques are available to ameliorate these effects. Since this is a rapidly evolving field of research, it is probable that new and important research will become available during the time it takes to bring this book to market. A revised edition of this book will most likely be necessary in several years.

This book attempts to reach several types of readers. First, I hope it will be read by architects and engineers involved in building design, environmental-health practitioners concerned with the health effects of indoor air pollutants, and government officials at various levels involved with the regulatory aspects of the indoor air environment. In addition, I would like to reach the concerned citizen who wants to learn more about particular issues; for example, many office workers and homeowners have a lively interest in the potential health effects of breathing other people's cigarette smoke or of being exposed to formaldehyde emitted from urea-formaldehyde foam insulation. Another topic that many readers will probably find of interest is that of choosing appropriate control techniques for various pollutants.

The scope of research on indoor air pollution is wide and ever-changing. It is not possible to cover all areas of research in detail in one book of this size. Readers who wish to delve deeper into any topic are referred to the Sources and Suggested Reading for each chapter, at the end of the book. There are many more journal articles and reports available than can be referenced here, but those that are cited provide an entrée into the literature.

The sources referred to in this book were selected to illustrate particular points. In many cases, numerous articles illustrate the same point. I trust that researchers will not feel slighted if their work is not discussed, since what the book offers is not a literature review but rather a balanced discussion of the issues of indoor air pollution.

In order to reach a wide audience with diverse backgrounds, it was necessary to explain some concepts and define some terms that are well known to some readers of this book. I hope that this has been done without either irritating the knowledgeable or mystifying the newcomer. On the other hand, I have decided not to define such terms as hydrocarbons and nitrogen oxides in the text but to reserve such definitions for the Glossary.

Several readers reviewed the manuscript and offered suggestions, noted omissions, or discovered inaccuracies. These people are Dorothy Dickey and William Nazaroff of Lawrence Berkeley Laboratory; Ken Sexton, Director of the Indoor Air Quality Program at the Department of Health Services, State of California; Dr. John Spengler of the Harvard School of Public Health; and Professor Frederick Shair of the California Institute of Technology.

My wife, Ellen Matthews, wrote part of Chapter 10 on legal aspects of indoor air pollution and also reviewed the entire manuscript, offering many helpful suggestions. Finally, several people at Stanford University Press offered encouragement and editing advice along the way, most notably Grant Barnes and William Carver. I want especially to thank Andrew Alden for suggesting many valuable editorial improvements.

I.T.

Contents

Tables

Figures

Indoor Air Quality
and Human Health

1

Introduction

On the average, North Americans and Europeans spend 80 to 90 percent of their time indoors; thus, the air we breathe is mostly indoor air. Although that may appear to be obvious, until recent years most health studies did not take this fact into account. In the past, studies concerned with the effects of air pollutants on human health considered only the exposure to outdoor pollutants, but indoor pollutants are a distinct and diverse group of their own.

In order to understand the effects of airborne substances on human health, it is important to know how much time people spend both outdoors and indoors, and also the concentrations of the pollutants to which they are exposed. Working people divide their time between home and work, while homemakers spend as much as 85 percent of their time at home. At home, people smoke, cook, paint, clean, heat the air for comfort, and carry out many other activities that can add harmful substances to the indoor air. The house itself, even the soil beneath it, can be a source of indoor air contaminants. Table 1.1 summarizes the main sources of indoor air pollutants and the contaminants they emit. Note that not all of these contaminants come from indoor sources.

Awareness of indoor air quality could be said to be a child of the 1973 oil embargo, for with that event came the surge of energy-conserving practices and devices that had a direct effect on the nation's indoor air. Making machines run more efficiently and designing furnaces to waste less heat are entirely beneficial actions, but putting certain types of insulation in houses, reducing ventilation in office buildings, and stopping drafts by "tightening" homes had unexpected side effects: indoor air pollution–related complaints began to increase as pollutants were kept bottled up

Table 1.1. Summary of Sources and Types of Indoor Air Pollutants

Sources	Pollutant types
Outdoor	
Stationary sources	Sulfur dioxide, ozone, particulates, carbon monoxide, hydrocarbons
Motor vehicles	Carbon monoxide, lead, nitrogen oxides
Soil	Radon, microorganisms
Indoor	
Building construction materials	
Concrete, stone	Radon
Particle board, plywood	Formaldehyde
Insulation	Formaldehyde, fiberglass
Fire retardant	Asbestos
Paint	Organics, lead
Building contents	
Heating and cooking combustion appliances	Carbon monoxide, nitrogen oxides, formaldehyde, particulates
Copy machines	Ozone, organics
Water service	Radon
Human occupants	
Metabolic activity	Carbon dioxide, water vapor, odorants
Biological activity	Microorganisms
Human activities	
Tobacco smoking	Carbon monoxide, particulates, odorants
Aerosol sprays	Fluorocarbons, odorants
Cleaning	Organics, odorants
Hobbies and crafts	Organics, odorants

indoors for longer periods of time. It should be noted that not all indoor air quality problems are a result of energy-efficiency improvements.

Several of these pollutants are of great importance and appear frequently in the news. Although our knowledge is still incomplete, the consensus is that three contaminants deserve the most intense study: (1) radon, a natural radioactive gas, (2) formaldehyde, a widely used chemical that emanates from many household items, and (3) tobacco smoke. The health effects involved range from eye and throat irritation through asthma and chronic respiratory disease to lung cancer.

These three do not exhaust the list. Residential kerosene heaters have dangers known and not-so-well known. Schools and offices may subject their occupants to asbestos-laden air. Many modern, airtight offices have been subject to epidemics of "tight-building syndrome." Utility-sponsored programs to weatherize houses, if not done carefully, may have unexpected impacts on customers' health. Finally, there are the spectacular outbreaks of illnesses such as Legionnaire's disease. This book provides the most up-to-date information for each of these issues, including ways to control exposure to contaminants indoors.

Exposures and Standards

Two factors that must be assessed in order to predict health effects are exposure levels and typical human responses for various levels of exposure. The type of exposure meant here is an *integrated* exposure, that is, the mathematical product of a pollutant concentration a person is exposed to and the time period over which the exposure occurs. Because the concentrations of pollutants that an individual is exposed to over the course of a day are often highly variable, the job of determining integrated exposures can be very difficult. Exposures may be acute (high concentrations for short time periods) or chronic (low concentrations for long time periods). Adverse health effects can be produced by either type of exposure.

For some airborne pollutants, the health effects of short-term exposures are well known. Data are often lacking, however, for long-term exposures to low concentrations of pollutants as experienced by occupants of residential and commercial buildings. The effect of a pollutant is often expressed in the form of a dose-response relationship. The *response* may range from eye irritation or headaches to lung cancer or death. For most of the pollutants we consider, the *dose* can be thought of as the amount of contaminant inhaled and reaching a particular part of the body; the dose is thus dependent upon the integrated exposure, the rate at which the individual takes in air, and the body's clearance rate for each contaminant. It is important to keep in mind that individuals vary in their respiratory rates and in their responses to various contaminants.

The federal government's efforts to monitor and improve air quality have concentrated on measuring pollutant concentrations in outdoor air and on controlling sources of outdoor air pollution. Because of this emphasis, there are large gaps in our knowledge of the integrated exposures to air pollutants experienced by various segments of the population. For example, we know comparatively little about the characteristics and concentrations of pollutants that homemakers, young children, and infirm adults are exposed to at home; neither are office workers a well-studied group. There are, however, a substantial number of studies from which we can make inferences about the range of exposures experienced by these groups given specific assumptions.

Once typical exposures are determined, health effects can be estimated for some pollutants. In this book we compare typical pollutant exposures to either dose-response relationships or to government health standards. These two approaches are often equivalent, since in most cases the health standards are derived from analysis of dose-response relationships. The health standards we refer to are those established by the Occupational

Table 1.2. National Primary Air Quality Standards

	Long-term		Short-term	
Contaminant	Concentration (ppm)	Averaging time (years)	Concentration (ppm)	Averaging time (hours)
Sulfur oxides	0.03	1	0.14	24
Carbon monoxide	—	—	9.0	8
	—	—	35.0	1
Ozone	—	—	0.12	1
Nitrogen dioxide	0.05	1	—	—
Particulates	75.0[a]	1	260.0	24

[a]Measured in micrograms per cubic meter ($\mu g/m^3$).

Safety and Health Administration (OSHA) and the Environmental Protection Agency (EPA). Although these health standards were not promulgated to apply to residential or office environments, they may be so used where the criteria they were based on are reasonable for that environment.

The Clean Air Act of 1970 directed the EPA to establish national standards for ambient air quality, which has thus far been interpreted to mean outdoor air. In 1971 the EPA announced final publication of national air quality standards for several classes of pollutants, including particulate matter, carbon monoxide, photochemical oxidants (mainly ozone), and nitrogen oxides. Although EPA standards apply to outdoor air, they were promulgated to protect the health of individuals of all ages, healthy or infirm. Therefore, assuming that the standards were soundly arrived at, for our purpose they can often be applied, with care, to indoor situations.* In particular, we will refer to the standards for ozone, carbon monoxide, and nitrogen oxides when attempting to predict the health effects resulting from indoor exposures to these pollutants. Indoor particulates, however, may be quite different from outdoor particulates: for example, tobacco-smoke particulates, often found indoors, are generally more harmful than the particulates found in outdoor air (such as ash, pollen, and soil).

Table 1.2 lists the EPA air quality standards. For some contaminants, such as carbon monoxide, there are two standards. A higher concentration is permissible for a shorter time period. The average carbon monoxide concentration for an 8-hour averaging period may not exceed 9 ppm (parts per million); for a 1-hour time period, however, the permissible concentration may go as high as 35 ppm.

A concentration of 35 ppm of carbon monoxide in air means that 35 of

*Since it was usually assumed that knowledge of the outdoor concentrations of the regulated pollutants was sufficient to determine exposures to population groups studied, actual and estimated exposures will vary for some pollutants. The criteria used to establish any standard must be assessed in order to determine its applicability to indoor air environments.

every million molecules in a sample of air are carbon monoxide molecules. Concentrations of gases can also be expressed in micrograms per cubic meter, a mass density. Particulate concentrations are always given as a mass density; that is, as a quantity of mass (often expressed in grams) that is found in some volume of air (for example, a cubic meter).

The occupational standards established by OSHA are designed to protect the health of most workers who are exposed to hazardous chemicals only during a 40-hour work week. They were intended to be applied to industrial environments. Office workers fall in a gray area, since they belong to the category of workers, but their activities are not carried out in an industrial environment. The National Institute of Occupational Safety and Health (NIOSH), a research arm of OSHA, and some state public health departments have been investigating indoor air problems in office buildings and, for lack of more applicable standards, have been applying OSHA standards. In this book, the most appropriate health standard will be chosen for determining health effects of a pollutant.

Air Infiltration

Substances emitted into the indoor air have much less opportunity to become diluted than those emitted outdoors, where there is a large volume of air available to disperse pollutants. The indoor concentration of any contaminant is determined by its rate of emission into the indoor space and its rate of removal from that space. The two processes that increase indoor contaminant concentrations are the flow of outdoor contaminants into the interior and the emission of contaminants from indoor sources; the two processes that decrease indoor contaminant levels are the flow of indoor air to the outside and the removal of contaminants by physical and chemical processes within the indoor environment. Removal may occur, for example, when particulate matter in the air becomes attached to walls or is trapped in the filter of an air-cleaning device. (Appendix A presents a theoretical mass-balance model that gives these processes exact expression.)

In residential buildings, indoor air contaminants are most commonly removed by dilution with outside air that leaks inside. As long as the concentration of the contaminant in question is lower outdoors than indoors, air exchange between outside and inside air will lower its indoor concentration. Of course, if a contaminant has an outdoor source but no indoor sources, air exchange will increase its indoor concentration; for example, in cities where photochemical smog is prevalent, the concentration of ozone is usually higher outside buildings.[1] Therefore, bringing in more outside air would raise the indoor ozone concentration.

Buildings that have low rates of air exchange with the outside air are

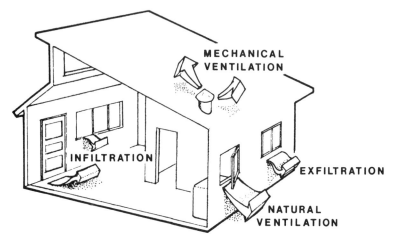

Fig. 1.1. Pathways of air exchange. Infiltration and exfiltration occur through cracks in the building envelope. Natural ventilation occurs through open doors and windows. Mechanical ventilation uses fans to force the movement of air. Source: *Indoor Air Quality Handbook* (Albuquerque, NM: Sandia National Laboratories and AnaChem, Inc., 1982).

often designated as tight or energy-efficient. They are energy-efficient because less cold air leaks into the building in the winter, decreasing the energy needed to heat this cold air to room temperature and thus reducing the cost of heating. In hot weather, less energy is used for air conditioning.

The uncontrolled leakage of outside air into a building is known as *infiltration*. Pressure differences, resulting from both wind and temperature differences between inside and outside air, force air through openings in the building's exterior. Air enters through cracks and leaky joints in the exterior walls, around doors, windows, and chimneys, and through other openings (see Fig. 1.1). Air also enters through open doors and windows in the process called *natural ventilation*. When a fan is used to bring air into a building, the process is designated as *forced ventilation*.

The leakiness of buildings may be compared by measuring their infiltration rates, as expressed by air changes per hour. One air change per hour means that a volume of air equal to the house volume leaks in from the outside each hour; correspondingly, an equal amount of inside air leaks out each hour. The infiltration rate of any building does not remain constant but is found to vary with wind velocity and inside-outside temperature difference. Residential buildings have average infiltration rates ranging from 0.2 to 2.0 air changes per hour (ach). Most conventionally built houses have average infiltration rates of 0.6 to 1.2 ach. A house of

1,500 square feet with a ceiling height of 8 feet has a volume of 12,000 cubic feet; 1 ach in this house is equivalent to 200 cubic feet per minute (cfm) of air exchange between inside and outside.

All other things being equal, the concentration of indoor-generated pollutants will be higher in houses with low infiltration rates if the indoor pollutant sources are of similar magnitude in the buildings being compared. Of course, even a high infiltration rate will not ensure good air quality if the sources are strong. In addition, it should be kept in mind that a high outdoor concentration of pollutants will lead to high indoor concentrations of those same pollutants when the infiltration rate is high. Except in particularly smoggy areas, all other factors being equal, looser homes will generally have lower indoor concentrations of air contaminants than tightly constructed homes. However, looser homes are less energy-efficient. Chapter 7 will consider the conflict between energy efficiency and indoor air quality in greater detail.

Outdoor Air as a Source of Indoor Air Pollution

When polluted outdoor air enters a building, it becomes a source of indoor air pollution. Pollutants can infiltrate a building's exterior along with the air that carries them, but measurements have shown that a building's envelope (walls, windows, and roof) acts as a screen to many outdoor air pollutants, and concentrations of sulfur dioxide, nitrogen dioxide, and ozone are lower indoors than outdoors where indoor sources of these pollutants are absent.[2]

The composition of outside air varies from one location to another, and depends upon the nature of the air pollution sources in the vicinity and the prevailing wind direction. Although the atmosphere is composed of a large number of gases, five of them (nitrogen, oxygen, argon, carbon dioxide, and water vapor) make up 99.99 percent of it by volume. Table 1.3 gives the average composition of dry air, in addition to which there may be significant quantities of water vapor and suspended particulates.

These concentrations can also be expressed in parts per million; for ex-

Table 1.3. Average Composition of the Atmosphere Below 15 Miles, Excluding Water Vapor

Component	Percent of total volume	Component	Percent of total volume
Nitrogen	78.08%	Neon	0.00180%
Oxygen	20.94	Helium	0.00052
Argon	0.93	Methane	0.00013
Carbon dioxide	0.032	Ozone	0.000002

ample, the natural background concentrations of carbon dioxide and ozone are approximately 320 ppm and 0.02 ppm respectively. If there are no major sources of these gases in the outdoor air sampled, then these are the concentrations that would be generally found. Other pollutants to be discussed later are present naturally in very small amounts: carbon monoxide, 0.1 ppm; nitric oxide, 0.003 ppm; and nitrogen dioxide, 0.001 ppm. In polluted urban air, the concentrations of all of these contaminants are higher.

There are three main sources of manmade air pollutants in the outdoor air: fuel combustion in stationary sources (such as power plants), fuel combustion in mobile sources (such as automobiles), and industrial processes (such as oil refining). The five main categories of air pollutants emitted by these sources are carbon monoxide, sulfur oxides, nitrogen oxides, hydrocarbons, and particulates. Fuel combustion in vehicles is the main source of carbon monoxide and hydrocarbons, and a major source of nitrogen oxides. Fuel combustion in stationary sources is the main source of sulfur oxides. Industrial processes and stationary combustion sources account for more than half of the particulates emitted into the air through human activities. There are also natural sources of particulates such as volcanic dust, eroded soil particles, spores and microbes, and wind-blown sea salt.

Determining Health Effects

When the EPA set air quality standards to protect people from the adverse health effects of exposure to airborne pollutants, two types of data were available, epidemiological and toxicological. Because these two ways to study health effects are the basis of this book's advice, it will be useful to discuss the general strategy and limitations of these approaches.

Toxicology is defined as the study of poisons; however, a toxicologist often works with substances we don't normally think of as poisons, such as food additives or air pollutants. Ideally, a toxicologist would like to know all of the effects of a known dose of a substance on humans. As discussed earlier, for airborne pollutants the dose is determined from the integrated exposure and the respiration rate of an individual. Other important factors in determining health effects are the absorption, detoxification, and excretion rates for each pollutant at different body sites. Rather than determine each of these factors, the responses to known exposures are usually studied by administering the substance in known amounts to animals or human volunteers. The data obtained can be summarized in a dose-response curve (see Fig. 1.2).

The toxicologist concentrates on a few major questions: Is there a threshold or minimum dose required before the effect of interest is mani-

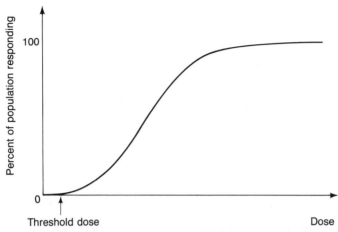

Fig. 1.2. A dose-response curve shows what percent of a population will have a particular response to a known dose of a physical, chemical, or biological agent. Few people respond to small doses, but most or all people respond to large doses.

fested? Is the substance toxic only when large doses are given in a short time (days or weeks); that is, what is its *acute toxicity*? Is it toxic when small doses are given over a period of years; that is, what is its *chronic toxicity*? Finally, which tests on animals can be extrapolated to humans?

Short-term responses a toxicologist looks for include changes in respiratory rate or keenness of perception, psychological effects, or diseases of various kinds. Some of the long-term effects usually looked for are cancer, birth defects, and alteration of genetic material. An example of a toxicological study for which a dose-response curve might be prepared is a test of the curative power of a new drug. The drug is administered to rats with a respiratory illness, and the number of rats cured is recorded. At small doses of the drug, no rats are cured. At higher doses (the threshold dose), some rats are cured, and at very high doses (if the drug is safe), almost all rats are cured.

Epidemiological studies generally begin with the effect and work back to probable causes by analyzing the health histories and habits of groups of people living in some community. Such studies have the advantage of examining illness where it occurs naturally, rather than in a laboratory, but they cannot control precisely all the factors of possible importance. Most epidemiological research deals with tests of association, and a single study can almost never be interpreted as proving causation. For example, an epidemiological study might show that there is a very strong association between cigarette smoking and lung cancer (which is the case), but it cannot prove in a scientific sense that cigarette smoking causes lung cancer. There are other causes of lung cancer, such as exposure to industrial pollutants and radiation. A conclusion from a hypothetical study might read as follows: The probability that a person who smokes a pack of cigarettes a day (over some time period) will contract lung cancer is ten times that for a nonsmoker. Epidemiological and toxicological studies are statistical in nature and always deal with probabilities.

A difficult problem faced by epidemiologists is determining an average exposure to a pollutant to be assigned to all members of a population, given that the concentration of various pollutants varies with time and location. In order to obtain a person's total exposure to a chemical, it would be necessary to have a time history of their daily movements and knowledge of the concentration in air of that chemical at all locations, preferably at the breathing zone. Ideally, a personal air monitor should be carried around at all times.

Many factors affect human illness aside from the pollutant being studied. Epidemiologists try to eliminate the effects of as many of these factors as possible by choosing two population groups to study that are similar in terms of such factors as median age, sex ratio, social status, racial composition, cigarette smoking, and so forth, but different in terms of exposure to some pollutant. The list of factors affecting health status, unfortunately, is staggering; therefore, it is always possible to criticize epidemiological studies by saying that the association that is claimed to exist is really due to some variable that was not considered or that is not equal in the two groups. Nevertheless, carefully planned and executed epidemiological studies are still useful, especially when considered along with toxicological data for the same pollutant.

The Respiratory System

This introduction should not skip the lungs. The main function of the respiratory system is to provide oxygen to the cells of the body and to remove excess carbon dioxide from them. In addition, the respiratory system can carry other substances found in inhaled air. Gaseous and particulate airborne pollutants enter the human body mainly via the respiratory system. Damage to the respiratory organs may follow directly, or the pollutant may be transported in the blood to remote tissues or a susceptible organ of the body.

The respiratory system (Fig. 1.3) can be broken down into three parts for a clearer description: the nasopharyngeal structure, the conducting division, and the respiratory division. Air inhaled through the nose is warmed and moistened before it passes through the conducting division. The tubes of the conducting division (trachea and bronchioles) carry air to the lungs. The walls of these tubes are lined with mucus glands and

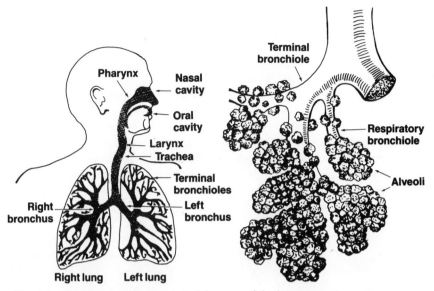

Fig. 1.3. Left, the major anatomical features of the human respiratory system. *Right*, the terminal bronchial and alveolar structure of the human lung. Source: *Air Quality Criteria for Particulate Matter*, National Air Pollution Control Association Publication no. AP-49.

hair cells, or cilia, that slowly transport particles up to the throat. The respiratory division begins with the respiratory bronchioles, which are small branches off the terminal bronchioles, and ends with the little air sacs called alveoli. It is here that oxygen and carbon dioxide are exchanged between air and blood. Air comes into intimate contact with the blood flowing through the capillaries, and the two gases are exchanged. Carbon dioxide is released from the blood to the lungs, and oxygen is transferred from the lungs to the blood. Tiny particles that reach the alveoli may be absorbed into the bloodstream; they may be engulfed by macrophages, a type of white blood cell; or they may remain in the alveoli, possibly exerting toxic effects if they contain asbestos or nicotine, for example.

Plan of the Book

This book attempts to cover the field of indoor air quality by starting simply—but even the simple things have their complications. Chapter 2 treats gaseous chemical contaminants, formaldehyde in particular. Chapter 3 addresses radon, a radioactive gas that decays into several radioactive substances that can cause lung cancer if inhaled. Particulate matter, the subject of Chapter 4, includes a great variety of substances and health effects, some of which involve the pollutants of earlier chapters. Chapter 5, on combustion products, takes a close look at the everyday activities of heating and cooking; these have both hazards and remedies.

The problem of involuntary smoking, surveyed in Chapter 6, touches on each previous chapter and adds to them the legal battles going on in this very personal controversy. The law has had its hand, too, in promoting energy-efficient houses, which as Chapter 7 shows may have unhealthy side effects. After all these problems, a survey of solutions, presented in Chapter 8, is in order. Chapter 9 examines the peculiar problems of the modern, airtight office buildings so many people work in. Finally, Chapter 10 is a primer on the legal doctrines that bear on indoor air pollution and an introduction to the government agencies whose regulations impinge on indoor air.

2

Formaldehyde and Other Household Contaminants

At great expense, Michael Wagner of Bayville, New Jersey, had his house torn apart. He paid $20,000 to have the new insulation removed from the walls of his house because it made him and his family sick. Shortly after the insulation was installed, Wagner began having equilibrium problems, severe headaches, and nosebleeds; his capacity to handle stress dwindled. "Eventually I collapsed at work and had to be rushed to the emergency room," he recalled during a television interview.[1] After health officials pinpointed formaldehyde emanating from the insulation as the probable cause of the family's symptoms, Wagner sued the manufacturer and the installer, who settled out of court for $225,000. The Wagners had suffered from formaldehyde sensitization.

The Wagners' case was extreme but not rare. Modern life has brought us into contact with thousands of chemical products; not surprisingly, dozens of them, some of which are listed in Table 2.1, can be significant polluters of the air at home or work. Formaldehyde, the most widespread and well known of these, has been the cause of thousands of complaints to the Consumer Product Safety Commission.

All of the substances mentioned in this chapter share some distinctive characteristics. As gases, they can bypass the lungs' defenses easily; those that dissolve in water readily enter the bloodstream. Some can penetrate the skin directly. They are all relatively immune to physical treatments like screens and filters. Countering them requires measures to prevent their formation, contain their release, or disperse them quickly.

Several other gaseous hazards are treated in separate chapters. Radon is one, a radioactive gas emitted by soil, stone, and other natural building materials but not limited to these sources. Combustion gases from space heating appliances and tobacco smoke are others.

Table 2.1. Sources of Formaldehyde and Other Household Air Contaminants

Source	Pollutant
Particle board, plywood, carpets, UF foam insulation	Formaldehyde
Aerosol sprays	Nitrous oxide, methylene chloride
Paint	Benzene, toluene, other organics
Plastics, synthetic rubber	Styrene
Solvents	Xylene, toluene, benzene, other organics
Cleaning products	Ammonia, chlorine, organics
Pesticides	Chlordane, pentachlorophenol

Formaldehyde Sources

A colorless gas with a characteristic pungent odor, formaldehyde is primarily an indoor-generated pollutant; its sources are building materials, insulation, furniture, carpets, combustion appliances, tobacco smoke, and various consumer products. Eight billion pounds of formaldehyde are produced in the United States each year. It is found in cosmetics, deodorants, solvents, disinfectants, and fumigants.

Urea-formaldehyde (UF) resin, which is produced from a mixture of urea, formaldehyde, and water, is the most common adhesive used in plywood, particle board, and chipboard. Plywood is composed of several thin sheets of wood glued together with UF resin; particle board and chipboard are made by impregnating wood chips or sawdust with UF resin and pressing the mixture into the final form. Emissions from UF-bonded chipboard and particle board are due to unreacted formaldehyde that remains in the product after manufacture, and also to the subsequent breakdown of the resin by its reaction with moisture and heat.

Urea-formaldehyde foam has been used extensively as thermal insulation in the walls of existing residential buildings. It is injected into wall cavities through small holes that are sealed afterwards. Installation involves mixing UF resin with a foaming agent and compressed air; the resulting product has the consistency of shaving cream. In typical applications, the foam is pumped through a hose and forced into the wall cavity, where it quickly cures and hardens.

Urea-formaldehyde foam was developed in Germany in the 1930's. By the early 1960's, UF foam was a common insulation material in northern Europe. It is effective insulation, as shown in Table 2.2 by its high R-value; however, it has been known to shrink over time, leaving it with a resistance value no higher than other types of insulation listed in the table. After limited safety studies, UF foam was approved for home insulation in the United States in the early 1970's. The rapid rise in prices for home heating fuels prompted many homeowners to install UF foam in

Table 2.2. R-Values for Insulation Materials
(Inches)

R-value	Glass fiber	Rock wool	Cellulose fiber	UF foam[a]
R-11	3.5	3.0	3.0	2.9
R-19	6.0	5.0	5.0	4.5
R-26	8.0	7.0	7.0	6.2
R-38	12.0	10.5	10.0	9.0

[a]The R-value for UF foam may be overestimated, owing to shrinkage after installation.

their walls. The process is fast, convenient for residents, and relatively cheap for existing homes. Blanket or batt-type insulation cannot be installed in existing buildings without removing the exterior or interior walls.

The amount of formaldehyde gas released from UF foam insulation depends on many factors, including the quality and age of ingredients, the proportion and mixing of ingredients, and the expertise of the installer. Even proper formulation and mixing of UF foam will not entirely prevent some formaldehyde release. High temperatures, as may occur when the sun is shining on a wall with UF foam inside, may cause the foam to deteriorate, thus liberating formaldehyde.

General Health Effects and Standards for Formaldehyde

Formaldehyde is a water-soluble gas that can be detected by most people at levels well below 1 ppm. Connecting specific health effects to specific concentrations of formaldehyde is difficult because people vary widely in their responses and complaints. Furthermore, an individual may become sensitized as a result of repeated exposure to formaldehyde. This is demonstrated by the higher frequency of dermatitis and asthma in the occupants of UF-foam-insulated houses.

Formaldehyde toxicity is brought about by contact with skin and the mucous membranes of the eyes, nose, and throat. Exposure to formaldehyde may cause burning eyes and irritation of the upper respiratory passages at concentrations as low as 0.05 ppm in sensitive individuals under certain conditions of temperature and humidity. Table 2.3 summarizes the reported health effects of formaldehyde at various concentrations derived from a report by the National Research Council Committee on Aldehydes.[2] Concentrations higher than a few parts per million often produce coughing, constriction in the chest, and wheezing. Over time, formaldehyde may cause chronic respiratory disease.

Studies in rats and mice have shown that concentrations of formaldehyde of several parts per million for several months induce nasal cancer.[3] This research, performed by the Chemical Industry Institute of Toxicology, found that rats exposed to 15 ppm of formaldehyde for 6 hours a day, 5 days a week, contracted nasal cancer after 11 months of exposure. Rats exposed to 2 and 6 ppm of formaldehyde developed structural changes in their nasal mucous membranes. These tissues, through the secretion of mucus and the action of cilia, clear foreign material from the nose. If this nasal defense system is disturbed, other noxious materials ordinarily cleared from the airways may be retained. Thus formaldehyde has both a direct and an indirect effect on the respiratory system.

The carcinogenic effects of formaldehyde exposure in humans have not been fully assessed. However, a recent epidemiological study by the Du Pont Corporation found no overall excess of cancer deaths in occupationally exposed persons compared with other nonexposed employees.[4] Adequate employee protection, it was claimed, was provided by maintaining exposure levels of 1 ppm as a time-weighted average and a 2-ppm ceiling limit.

There is no outdoor standard for formaldehyde in the United States, but the American Industrial Hygiene Association recommends a guideline of 0.1 ppm. The Netherlands, in 1978, established an indoor standard of 0.1 ppm maximum permissible concentration; Denmark, Sweden, and West Germany may all establish standards at approximately the same value. The present Occupational Safety and Health Administration standard for occupational exposure is 3 ppm for an 8-hour time-weighted average. The National Institute of Occupational Safety and Health is rec-

Table 2.3. Reported Health Effects of Formaldehyde
at Various Concentrations

Effects	Approximate concentration (ppm)
None reported	0.0–0.05
Odor threshold	0.05–1.0
Neurophysiologic effects [a]	0.05–1.5
Eye irritation	0.01–2.0[b]
Upper airway irritation	0.10–25
Lower airway and pulmonary effects	5.0–30
Pulmonary edema, inflammation, pneumonia	50–100
Death	100+

SOURCE: National Research Council, *Formaldehyde and Other Aldehydes* (Washington, DC: National Academy Press, 1981). By permission of the publisher.

[a] Changes in electroencephalograms and in the response of dark-adapted eyes to light.

[b] The response to 0.01 ppm occurred in the presence of other pollutants.

Table 2.4. Formaldehyde Standards

	Level (ppm)	Status
Outdoor air		
United States	0.1	Recommended by ACGIH[a]
Indoor air		
California	0.2	Proposed
	0.05 (new mobile homes)	Recommended
Minnesota	0.5	Proposed
Wisconsin	0.2	Effective
Denmark	0.12	Recommended
Netherlands	0.1	Effective
Sweden	0.1 (new buildings)	Proposed
	0.4–0.7 (old buildings)	Proposed
Germany	0.1	Proposed
Occupational air		
United States	3.0 (8-hr average)	Promulgated by OSHA
	5.0 (maximum)	Promulgated by OSHA
	2.0 (maximum)	Recommended by ACGIH[a]
	1.0 (30-min average)	Recommended by NIOSH

[a] American Conference of Governmental Industrial Hygienists.

ommending that this be strengthened to 1 ppm maximum for a 30-minute time period. Table 2.4 summarizes existing and proposed formaldehyde health standards. It appears that for the nonoccupational indoor environment, a consensus of 0.1 to 0.5 ppm of formaldehyde for a health standard has developed among many governmental regulatory agencies.

Health and Air Quality Surveys

Health studies of residential formaldehyde have generally concentrated either on houses with UF foam insulation or on mobile homes. In foam-insulated houses, the large surface area of the formaldehyde source is responsible for the high levels in the air. Mobile homes are prone to indoor air pollution of all kinds because they are built more airtight than houses; moreover, they commonly contain large amounts of particle board and plywood. However different the sources are, the health effects are similar.

A few studies have compared the concentration of formaldehyde in homes with UF foam insulation to those without it. In Canada, where UF foam has been banned, formaldehyde levels were measured in several thousand homes. Homes with UF foam had formaldehyde levels two to three times that in homes without it. (The Canadian government gives $5,000 to all homeowners with UF foam insulation to help defray the cost of replacing it.)

The Connecticut State Health Department surveyed 84 homes with UF foam insulation in which residents complained of adverse symptoms. Formaldehyde levels ranged from 0.50 to 10 ppm, with a mean concentration of 1.8 ppm.[5] More limited studies of complaints in Colorado, Wisconsin, and elsewhere have found that in UF-foam-insulated houses where occupants have complained of adverse health effects, formaldehyde concentrations are sufficient to cause eye, nose, and throat irritation in exposed individuals. A study of foam-insulated homes where there were no occupant complaints found an average concentration of formaldehyde of 0.13 ppm as compared to 0.03 ppm in homes without UF foam.

The National Institute of Occupational Safety and Health recommends that formaldehyde levels be maintained below 1 ppm over any 30-minute time period. This maximum allowable concentration applies to healthy workers exposed for only 40 hours a week; of course, people who live in such an environment would have larger exposures. The concern is greatest for children, the infirm, and the elderly.

A study of formaldehyde concentrations in 40 homes was recently concluded for the Consumer Product Safety Commission by the Oak Ridge National Laboratory.[6] Eleven of the homes had UF foam insulation installed in the walls. The highest formaldehyde levels were found in homes with UF foam insulation and in newly constructed homes. The formaldehyde levels varied on both a daily and seasonal basis and increased as much as 20 times with increasing temperature and humidity. The average formaldehyde concentration was 0.06 ppm; the range was from 0.02 to 0.5 ppm.

A more extensive analysis of formaldehyde levels in residential homes was carried out by a manufacturer of passive formaldehyde monitors.[7] Five thousand samples collected and analyzed over a 6-month period throughout the United States showed that 58 percent of the homes had formaldehyde concentrations less than 0.05 ppm, 27 percent had concentrations ranging from 0.05 to 0.10 ppm, and 15 percent had concentrations greater than 0.10 ppm. This was probably not a random sample of residential buildings, because homeowners suspecting problems would be more likely to utilize the services of this manufacturer.

Over a 4-month period the Rocky Mountain Poison Center in Denver, Colorado, received complaints from more than 100 occupants of homes insulated with UF foam. About half of these people were studied by Dr. John Harris and his colleagues at the University of Colorado Health Sciences Center.[8] Only 38 percent of the occupants could smell the formaldehyde in their homes, which is consistent with the phenomenon of adaptation to odors. As Table 2.5 shows, almost half of the occupants experienced difficulty in breathing, headaches, and eye and nasal irritation; frequent colds were reported nearly as much. The average duration of the symptoms recorded was almost 14 months at the time of the study. More

Table 2.5. Frequency of Symptoms Reported
in 48 Occupants of Homes Insulated with UF Foam

Symptom	Percent of occupants	Symptom	Percent of occupants
Dyspnea[a]	46%	Frequent colds	38%
Headache	44	Rash	17
Rhinitis	44	Malaise	15
Eye irritation	40	Sore throat	6
Cough	40	Vomiting	4

SOURCE: J. C. Harris *et al.*, "Toxicology of Urea-Formaldehyde and Polyurethane Foam Insulation," *Journal of the American Medical Association*, vol. 245, no. 3 (January 1981). Copyright 1981, American Medical Association.
[a]Dyspnea is difficult and labored breathing.

troubling problems arose in some people: two cases of prolonged vomiting occurred in infants less than a year old.

There are over 4 million mobile homes in the United States. In general, mobile homes are built more tightly than conventional houses, which means there is less air exchange between outside and inside air. Indoor-generated pollutants can thus reach higher concentrations.

There have been many cases of persons living in mobile homes becoming sick in that indoor environment. The Consumer Products Safety Commission has documented over 1,000 complaints from mobile home owners reporting symptoms of formaldehyde exposure. Particle board seems to be the culprit in mobile homes: the floors and most of the cabinets in the kitchen and bathroom are made of it. Furniture is also often made of particle board.

Professor Peter Breysse, of the University of Washington School of Public Health, conducted a detailed study of 334 mobile homes in which one or more inhabitants complained of health problems.[9] Formaldehyde concentrations were measured once each in two locations within the home. Table 2.6 summarizes the results. The highest reading was 1.77 ppm, the lowest was 0.03 ppm. Of the 608 samples taken, two-thirds were between 0.1 and 0.5 ppm and one-fifth were greater than 0.5 ppm. Thus most of the people living in these homes were exposed to formaldehyde levels great enough to irritate the eyes and upper airways. Conventional homes typically have average formaldehyde readings below 0.07 ppm.

The researchers surveyed 523 occupants of these mobile homes: 240 women, 184 men, and 99 children (under 19 years of age). The most common symptoms were eye irritation (58 percent of the adults, 41 percent of the children) and throat irritation (66 percent of the adults, 62 percent of the children). One-third of the children experienced chronic cough or cold symptoms. About half of the adults reported chronic headache and over 20 percent complained of memory lapse or drowsiness.

Table 2.6. Formaldehyde Concentrations in Mobile Homes
with Occupant Complaints

Concentration	Kitchen	Bedroom	Other room	Total
>1.0 ppm	7	7	2	16
0.5–0.99 ppm	53	44	15	112
0.1–0.49 ppm	198	161	48	407
<0.1 ppm	34	36	3	73
TOTAL	292	248	68	608

SOURCE: P. A. Breysse, *Formaldehyde Exposure in Mobile Homes* (Seattle: University of Washington, School of Public Health, 1980). By permission of the author.

These results came from a group of people with acknowledged health problems, and though they cannot be generalized to all mobile home owners, the numbers are suggestive. Moreover, Breysse found that all the occupants complaining of health effects experienced relief whenever they left their homes on weekends or vacations. Proof is seldom perfect in science, but the set of facts Breysse uncovered points to formaldehyde as the causative agent.

Another finding was that those who had suffered over long periods of time often developed acute depression. This may reflect the fact that many of the respondents to the survey were being treated by their doctors with no significant relief; a few were even accused of being hypochondriacs by their doctors or spouses.

Breysse pointed out that many of the people living in mobile homes are old and more infirm than the general population. These people are more susceptible to the adverse effects of formaldehyde because they have more allergies, emphysema, bronchitis, and heart disease.

Particle board is not limited to mobile homes, so it is no surprise that it causes problems elsewhere. In a housing project in Bloomington, Minnesota, more than 400 residents showed symptoms of formaldehyde exposure.[10] The problem was traced to particle-board shelving in the cabinets. Health officials found an average of 0.25 ppm of formaldehyde in the air of 120 units where complaints were registered. The particle board had been coated with sealing agents like shellac to reduce emissions, but that was clearly not sufficient. The state of Minnesota now requires all real-estate agents to warn buyers of new homes about the dangers of formaldehyde. New houses in Minnesota, like cigarette packs, may contain a warning that living here may be hazardous to your health.

Formaldehyde problems are known in other nations, too. In the Netherlands, many formaldehyde measurements have been made in houses, schools, and offices where chipboard was used.[11] Large amounts of chipboard made from ground wood and urea-formaldehyde glue were incorporated into inner walls, roof plates, ceilings, and furniture. Of 36 houses

Table 2.7. Highest Measured Concentrations of Formaldehyde in Dutch Houses

Location	Concentration (ppm)	Room with highest concentration
Oudenbosch[a]	0.25	Attic
Haarlem		
House 1	0.68	Bedroom
House 2	0.80	Bedroom
House 3	1.50	Hall
House 4	0.24	Living room
Drachten[a]	0.21	Bedroom
Nootdorp	0.48	Office/shop
Leeuwarden		
House 1	0.45	Bedroom
House 2	0.63	Bedroom
House 3	0.21	Bedroom
House 4	0.18	Bedroom
House 5	0.17	Living room
House 6	0.23	Attic
House 7	0.33	Attic
House 8	0.13	Attic
House 9	0.28	Bedroom
House 10	0.24	Living room
Emmen		
House 1	0.13	Bedroom
House 2	0.06	Bedroom
House 3	0.03	Bedroom
House 4	0.05	Bedroom
Schoonebeek	0.03	Bedroom
Diemen		
House 1	0.24	Attic (bedroom)
House 2	0.18	Attic (bedroom)
Lelystad		
House 1[b]	0.21	Study
House 2	0.27	Bedroom
Waddinxveen	0.13	Living room
Monster	0.19	Bedroom
Zaandam		
House 1	0.29	Bedroom
House 2	0.12	Attic (bedroom)
House 3	0.09	Bedroom
House 4	0.14	Attic (bedroom)
House 5	0.13	Bedroom
House 6	0.09	Bedroom
House 7	0.13	Bedroom
Stellendam	0.08	Attic

SOURCE: J. F. van der Wal, "Formaldehyde Measurements in Dutch Houses, Schools, and Offices," *Atmospheric Environment*, vol. 16, no. 10 (1982). By permission of the author.

[a] House not yet inhabited.
[b] Not inhabited; show house.

investigated (in all cases occupants complained to the health department), only 7 had a formaldehyde concentration below the limit of 0.1 ppm in all rooms. In 6 houses the concentration exceeded 0.4 ppm. Table 2.7 shows the highest concentration in each house investigated and the room where the highest concentration was found—usually the bedroom.

The Foam Ban

Although the Wagners' reaction to formaldehyde, described at the beginning of the chapter, is an extreme one, it is not that far from the examples discussed above. There have been thousands of consumer complaints received at the Consumer Product Safety Commission (CPSC) concerning health effects from the use of UF foam insulation. In February 1982, the CPSC voted to ban UF foam insulation as a hazardous consumer product, determining that it presents an unreasonable risk of acute and chronic illness because of the formaldehyde gas it releases and because the amount of formaldehyde that will be released from the product cannot be predicted. In many homes there is a low concentration of formaldehyde because the dangerous material is well sealed, and thus risk of injury to people living in these homes is reduced.

Industry groups such as the Formaldehyde Institute opposed the ban and challenged it in the courts. In 1983 a three-judge panel of the Fifth Circuit Court of Appeals ruled that the CPSC used faulty evidence in finding that UF foam insulation increased the risk of cancer and respiratory ailments. Although UF foam insulation may now be used, there is actually little, if any, being installed in residences and schools. The adverse publicity from the ban and numerous court actions have effectively stopped its use. However, there are over 500,000 homes in the United States and over 100,000 in Canada with UF foam insulation installed. Thousands of lawsuits have been filed for homeowners seeking damages from manufacturers and installers of UF foam insulation. A $2 billion class-action lawsuit was filed in 1982 on behalf of the 70,000 to 130,000 residents of New York State who have UF foam insulation installed in their homes.[12]

A Homeowner's Guide to Solving UF Foam Problems

The owner or resident of a house with UF foam insulation has a distinctive set of likely problems; each one has clear solutions, but some are drastic and expensive. Hence the need for this section, which should help homeowners sort out what they may need to do, or at least tell them whom to consult next.

The CPSC's ban has been overturned, but many people still have questions about the health effects of exposure to formaldehyde and about methods of reducing formaldehyde emissions from UF foam insulation. About a million people live in homes with UF foam insulation installed in their walls. Much of what follows is based on a memorandum prepared by the Consumer Product Safety Commission before the ban was overturned.[13]

The signs of exposure to formaldehyde vapors from UF foam insulation include eye, nose, and throat irritation, persistent cough, respiratory distress, skin irritation, nausea, headaches, and dizziness. The severity of these illnesses varies from short-term discomfort to serious impairment. Some persons have been hospitalized. Chronic respiratory problems such as asthma have resulted from exposure to formaldehyde gas, and existing respiratory illnesses have been made worse by it. Heavy doses of formaldehyde can cause cancer in rats. Thus, there may be some unknown low-level risk of cancer from formaldehyde exposure in the home.

A home insulated before 1970 probably does not have UF foam insulation. It may be possible to check with the builder, real estate agent, or seller to find out if foam insulation was ever installed. The insulation contractor may know, or the contract or bill of sale may say. If the insulation was blown in through holes in the walls, then it *may* be UF foam insulation—cellulose insulation is also blown in. If the insulation was not blown in, then it was not UF foam insulation. Sampling inside the walls will give the best answer.

Some local and state health departments conduct formaldehyde tests at no cost to residents; others charge a modest fee. If these sources are unavailable, a commercial laboratory may be able to determine the concentration of formaldehyde in the air. Companies that perform this service may be listed in the Yellow Pages under "laboratories." Three companies that sell measuring devices that can be used to determine formaldehyde levels are listed in Appendix B. Once the levels are known, the hazard can be assessed.

It is not possible to define a minimum level of formaldehyde that will rule out all adverse health effects. Less than 20 percent of healthy adults may react to formaldehyde at less than 0.25 ppm. Because people vary in their response to formaldehyde, any reaction and its severity will differ among people exposed to the same level of formaldehyde. Only one member of a family may suffer. Infants, those with allergies or respiratory problems, and the elderly may be more sensitive or respond more severely.

Most healthy adults may not experience acute toxic effects from formaldehyde exposure below 0.1 ppm, but some definitely do. Anyone experiencing symptoms that may be related to exposure to formaldehyde, regardless of the measured levels, should consult a doctor. While it is difficult to establish an exact level of concern, if the concentration of formaldehyde averaged over a 24-hour period is above 0.1 ppm, additional measurements may be in order to determine how formaldehyde levels change with time, temperature, and humidity.

If the occupants have not experienced any adverse health effects from their foam insulation, it may be that the formaldehyde gas is not entering the house in excessive amounts and, therefore, may not be a serious problem. On the other hand, they may not be very sensitive to formaldehyde on an *acute* basis. Since long-term health effects are possible, they may still wish to measure the formaldehyde concentration.

After learning the formaldehyde levels and seeing the doctor, there are several things to do. First, the affected occupants should try to follow their physician's advice, even if that advice is to move. Second, they should increase ventilation by opening windows when the weather permits. Third, they should contact the installer who foamed their house as well as the company that provided the chemicals to the installer. They should ask what corrective action the company and installer are prepared to take; if this is not enough to relieve the off-gassing problem, they can take some corrective actions on their own, as discussed below. Affected residents may also wish to seek assistance from their local government consumer affairs office. Finally, legal remedies may be pursued by bringing suit, if necessary, against the foam manufacturer and insulation installer.

The National Research Council of Canada (NRCC) has recommended techniques that offer some relief for owners of houses with UF foam insulation. The NRCC suggests that occupants seal the walls to prevent infiltration of formaldehyde. Some of the steps that may be taken include (1) repairing all holes, cracks, or gaps in the wall finish, using caulk or spackling compounds; (2) applying two coats of a vapor-barrier paint to the walls; and (3) laying mylar or vinyl wallpaper on the wall. Special paste and a good grade of canvas-backed vinyl wallpaper should be used. Both the paint and the vinyl wallpaper will not only seal in the formaldehyde but seal out moisture from the foamed wall. Walls that cannot be painted or papered can be varnished instead, and joints between panels sealed.

Painting and wallpapering are not necessarily enough. For example, electrical outlets may be filled in with UF foam, even if the insulation was properly installed. A cheap nonflammable gasket available at hardware stores may be installed under the cover plate to slow the flow of air and formaldehyde into the room. More important, however, is the junction of the wall and the floor where air can leak into the room. Here butyl or acrylic latex caulk, weatherstripping, or special foam-backed tapes can be used. The CPSC has no data from which to judge the effectiveness of these measures, although they are certainly effective to some degree.

Ammonia fumigation is a chemical method for reducing formaldehyde levels. In water solution, ammonia reacts readily with formaldehyde to form a stable chemical. Ammonium hydroxide is placed in shallow plastic pans in each major room, and the home is sealed for a minimum of 12 hours with the thermostat set at a minimum of 80°F. Precautions are taken to protect the person carrying out the fumigation, food, clothing, pets, house plants, and light-colored oak. The home is thoroughly ventilated with fans. According to tests by Weyerhaeuser Company, a residual ammonia odor disappears completely within several days.[14] Long-term reductions of formaldehyde levels by two-thirds have been claimed in mobile homes.

If the UF foam must be removed from the walls, the cost, according to the CPSC, can run from less than $5,000 to $20,000. The procedure involves removing interior and exterior wall panels or siding, removing the foam, and installing new insulation and wall panels or siding. Wood surfaces that come in contact with the foam are treated with a neutralizing chemical such as sodium bisulfite. This is a task for professionals.

Additional information on UF foam insulation may be obtained from the organizations listed in Appendix B.

Household Products

There are thousands of different household chemical products including detergents, soaps, oven cleaners, furniture polishes, paints, insecticides, glues, and so on, many of which come in the form of aerosol sprays. Many household products do not display a list of ingredients; thus consumers are often not aware of just what they are introducing to their indoor air. Because these products are used intermittently, it is very difficult to assess the overall health effects of their use. Though they are of great importance, the health effects of accidental ingestion of these chemicals will not be discussed in this book.

Table 2.8 lists some of the household products frequently used in residential buildings, and the pollutants released by them. The specific uses of these products, their ingredients, if known, and the health effects of these ingredients will be discussed below.

Aerosol Products

More than 40 aerosol spray products can be found in the average household during the course of a year. Aerosol containers are used to dis-

Table 2.8. Household Products and Pollutants Emitted

Product	Pollutants
Aerosol	Propane, nitrous oxide, methylene chloride
Household cleaners	Ammonia, chlorine
Furniture and floor polishes	Organics
Fresheners and disinfectants	Carbolic acid, cresol
Fabric-care products	Organics
Hobbies	Organics
Paint	Organics, heavy metals
Pesticides	Organics

pense a wide variety of products including pesticides, oven cleaners, deodorants, and paints. The containers hold three components: the active ingredient, the propellant, and miscellaneous additives used to improve the end product delivered. Common propellants used in aerosol spray cans are nitrous oxide and methylene chloride, both of which have an anesthetic effect on the central nervous system. When methylene chloride is inhaled it can undergo chemical change and be converted to carbon monoxide, which produces its own toxic effects on the body.

Cleaning Products

Household cleaning products of particular concern include oven cleaners, drain cleaners, and bleaches. Oven cleaners usually contain lye (sodium hydroxide) and other chemicals. Spray oven cleaner is the most hazardous type, since it disperses the chemical into the air where it may land on the skin or be inhaled. Lye is very irritating to the skin, eyes, and internal organs. Powdered oven cleaner is designed to release ammonia vapors when water is added. The fumes are noxious and dangerous to inhale in large quantities. Drain and toilet cleaners, which are close to 90 percent lye, do not present an indoor air quality problem when used alone. However, mixing chlorine bleach with drain or oven cleaners that contain ammonia produces chloramine, a deadly gas.

Air Fresheners and Disinfectants

Air fresheners usually work by masking bad odors with another aroma. A few air fresheners contain chemicals that diminish the ability to smell. The loss of the ability to smell, however temporary, can be not only sensually impoverishing but hazardous. Our noses let us detect fires at an early stage, toxic gases, and decayed food.

Disinfectants generally contain toxic chemicals such as cresol, which attacks the liver, kidneys, spleen, pancreas, and central nervous system; it may be absorbed through inhalation or through the skin.

Fabric Cleaners

Rug and upholstery cleaners and spot removers contain a wide variety of toxic chemicals. The former products are thought to contain the following ingredients: turpentine, borax, naphthalene, trichloroethane, and petroleum distillates (exact ingredients are trade secrets). Most of these compounds produce toxic fumes during use. Liquid spot removers contain trichloroethane, naphtha, ammonia hydroxide, benzene, toluene, and sodium hypochlorite. Again, the hazard associated with the use of spot removers is from fumes.

Hobbies

The major health effects arising from hobbies are due to inhalation, ingestion, and skin contact with toxic chemicals. Hobbies such as pottery, woodworking, sculpture, and metalworking generate airborne dust. Many glues and epoxy products are skin and lung irritants and are allergic sensitizers. Paint strippers used for refinishing furniture may contain toxic chemicals such as methylene chloride, a central nervous system depressant that is readily vaporized when used as a paint stripper.

Painting

Paints contain solvents that are released to the atmosphere as soon as they are exposed to the air. Toluene is one toxic chemical contained in paint. Toluene causes fatigue, muscle weakness, and confusion at concentrations of 200 to 300 ppm for 8 hours. When its vapors are inhaled, toluene causes central nervous system depression, psychosis, and liver and kidney damage. Toluene is also contained in glue and varnishes. Paint pigments may emit volatile toxic compounds containing lead, cadmium, mercury, and selenium.

When paints, varnishes, paint strippers, glues, and such are used indoors, it is very important to ventilate the work area much more than is typically done. Open doors and windows are needed. Better yet, do the work outdoors if possible.

Pesticides

Pesticides are commonly used in the home, garden, or lawn to kill various insects. Some are of special interest here.

Chlordane is frequently used on soil beneath wood structures to prevent termite damage to foundations. It has been discovered that chlordane vapor can penetrate openings in the undersides of buildings and reach the indoors. The symptoms reported include irritability and dizziness. Chlordane is a known animal carcinogen.

The pesticide pentachlorophenol (PCP) preserves wood, wood products, and glues. A 5 percent solution is used to preserve logs and redwood in homes constructed of wood. PCP continues to vaporize from treated wood even after seven years. In California and Kentucky, occupants of PCP-treated homes have become ill. The symptoms of exposure to PCP are corneal (eye) numbness, development of a blind spot, and autonomic nervous system impairment affecting such things as the heartbeat, sleep, and appetite. The widespread use and slow degradation of this pesticide raise concerns about its effects upon human health.

Volatile Organics

The 40-home study discussed earlier also included measurements of volatile organic compounds. Air samples were collected and studied by gas chromatography. From 20 to over 150 volatile organic compounds were observed in these homes, and in number and concentrations much greater indoors than outdoors. Table 2.9 lists those compounds that were

Table 2.9. Organic Compounds Commonly Found
in Residential Buildings

Compound	Winter mean (μg/m^3)	Summer mean (μg/m^3)
Toluene	27.2	61.7
Ethyl benzene	4.4	10.5
Xylene	16.6	44.2
Nonane	10.6	6.4
Cumene	2.2	1.3
Benzaldehyde	22.3	51.7
Mesitylene	1.4	6.7
Decane	12.4	8.9
Limonene	10.3	20.8
Undecane	8.2	12.0
Naphthalene	9.4	17.5
Dodecane	4.2	13.7
2-Methylnaphthalene	2.5	2.6
Tridecane	2.3	16.5
Tetradecane	3.2	7.5
Pentadecane	2.8	1.9
Hexadecane	3.7	3.8
Benzene	50.0	100.0

SOURCE: *Status Report on the Indoor Air Quality Monitoring Study in 40 Homes*, Oak Ridge National Laboratory (May 1984).

Table 2.10. Selected Organic Compounds and Their Health Effects

Compound	Health effects	Sources and uses
Formaldehyde and other aldehydes	Eye and respiratory irritation; possibly more-serious long-term health effects	Outgassing from building materials (particle board, plywood, and urea-formaldehyde insulation foam); also from cooking and smoking
Benzene	Respiratory irritation; recognized carcinogen	Plastic and rubber solvents; from cigarette smoking; in paints and varnishes, including putty, filler, stains, and finishes
Xylene	Narcotic; irritating; in high concentrations, possibly injurious to heart, liver, kidney, and nervous system	Solvent for resins, enamels, etc.; in non-lead automobile fuels and in manufacture of pesticides, dyes, pharmaceuticals
Toluene	Narcotic; may cause anemia	Solvents; by-product of organic compounds used in several household products
Styrene	Narcotic; can cause headache, fatigue, stupor, depression, incoordination, and possible eye injury	Widespread in manufacture of plastics, synthetic rubber, and resins
Trichloroethane	Subject of OSHA carcinogenesis inquiry	Aerosol propellant, pesticide, cleaning solvents
Trichloroethylene	Animal carcinogen; subject of OSHA carcinogenesis inquiry	Oil and wax solvents, cleaning compounds, vapor degreasing products, dry-cleaning operations; also as an anesthetic
Ethyl benzene	Severe irritation to eyes and respiratory system	Solvents; in styrene-related products
Chloro benzenes	Strong narcotic; possible lung, liver, and kidney damage	In production of paint, varnish, pesticides, and various organic solvents
Polychlorinated biphenyls (PCB's)	Suspected carcinogens	In various electrical components; in waste oil supplies and in plastic and paper products in which PCB's are used as plasticizers
Pesticides	Suspected carcinogens	Insect control

SOURCE: C. D. Hollowell and R. R. Miksch, *Sources and Concentrations of Organic Compounds in Indoor Environments*, Lawrence Berkeley Laboratory Report LBL-13195 (July 1981).

present most often in the test home and at higher levels than other organic compounds. The original analysis method did not allow measurement of the more highly volatile organics, such as aldehydes and halogenated hydrocarbons. Additional measurements suggested the presence of methylene chloride, trichloroethane, and perchloroethylene. Included among these chemicals and those listed in Table 2.9 are a human carcinogen (benzene), animal carcinogens, mutagens, and mucous membrane irritants. Table 2.10 lists the health effects of some common organic indoor air pollutants. At the low exposures experienced by most home occupants, the potential health effects of these volatile organic compounds are unknown; however, additional research in this area is certainly warranted.

3

Radon

Radioactive substances are different in many respects from other indoor air pollutants. The radiation they emit is invisible and odorless; and low-level exposure produces no immediate health effects such as headaches or eye irritation. There are no early warning signals that cancer may develop ten or twenty years after exposure.

We are always exposed to background radiation from natural sources, namely cosmic rays and radioactive elements in the earth's crust. It is likely that the small doses of radiation received by the general population have caused some disease and genetic change throughout history. But now that we live more of our lives indoors, one particular source has grown in importance: the radioactive gas called radon.

The Environmental Protection Agency has claimed that as many as 20,000 lung cancer deaths per year may result from exposure to radon and its radioactive decay products. This number is much higher than others put it, but as a worst-case estimate it will do for the discussions here. The deputy assistant administrator for radiation programs at the EPA, David Rosenbaum, has stated the threat as follows: "Radon is by far the highest radiation danger that the American public faces. It's certainly up there with the top dangers EPA deals with. It's easily more serious than Love Canal."[1]

Radon is a chemically inert, radioactive gas. It occupies a place in the radioactive decay series of uranium, the sets of subatomic reactions, well known to science, by which the heavy elements such as uranium and thorium change through many intermediate forms into lead. Radon is near the middle of the uranium series; it derives primarily from the radioactive decay of radium, and it decays, in turn, with a half-life of just under 4 days, through several more stages or daughter products, ending in lead. Some of these decay reactions emit alpha radiation—a fact of great importance for human health.

What makes all this information relevant is that radon is an inert gas. The other elements in the long cascade from uranium to lead are solids, and they are all chemically active. They stay locked up, for the most part, in the minerals where they form, and decay with little harm to anything else. By contrast, when a radium atom decays to radon it drifts, moving through the rocks and soil unattracted to other chemical elements. Some radon enters the air before it decays into its daughter products. The daughters in turn can become attached to particles in the air and lodge in the lungs if inhaled. There, they can cause damage to body tissue.

There are three important ways in which radon may enter buildings: by transport from soil through cracks and openings in the structure or around the foundation, through emanation from earth-derived building materials such as concrete, and by transport in water and natural gas (see Fig. 3.1). Soil is thought to be the major contributor to indoor radon in most U.S. houses, but some building materials may contain large amounts of radioactive substances. Phosphate slag was widely used from 1962 to 1977 as aggregate for the concrete foundation of homes built in southeastern Idaho.[2] In Sweden, many homes were constructed with a type of concrete that contained large amounts of radium.[3]

The concentration of radon in residences depends on several factors: the location of the building, the materials used to construct it, its foundation type, pathways for air transport from soil to basement, the source of its water supply, and the average ventilation rate. In parts of the United States and other countries (Sweden and Finland, for example) the soil and rocks are high in radium content. Stone, concrete, and brick emit radon, some more than others. A building's foundation type, by isolating the building from the underlying soil, may influence indoor radon concentrations: vented crawl spaces provide better ventilation than concrete slabs on grade or unvented basements, and thus may allow for more rapid dispersal of radon. Well water tends to have more dissolved radon than water from surface reservoirs. Finally, the ventilation rate is an important influence on the concentration of radon in a residence. All other things being equal, halving the ventilation rate will approximately double the radon concentration.

Radon concentrations are customarily much higher indoors than outdoors. The Lawrence Berkeley Laboratory has measured radon in more than 100 houses throughout the United States and found no clear correlation between radon concentrations and air infiltration rate. It is concluded that the observed differences in radon concentration reflect varia-

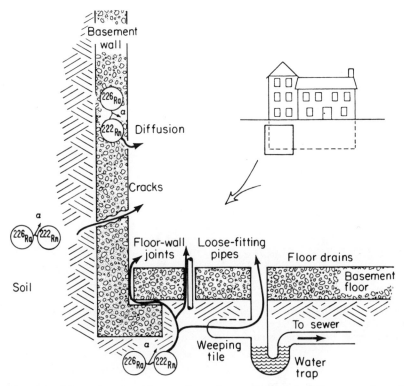

Fig. 3.1. The primary pathways for radon entry into buildings are through openings and cracks in foundations and by diffusion through the foundation walls and basement floor. Source: Lawrence Berkeley Laboratory.

tion from one house to another in the rate at which radon enters houses from its sources. Researchers believe that, in most cases, the soil beneath a house is the major source of radon.

Many people live in homes with radon-daughter concentrations that are much higher than the national average. Figure 3.2 illustrates the distribution of radon levels in homes in three locations, Sweden, Maine, and Texas.[4] The three histograms show the percentage of houses with radon levels in the range shown on the horizontal axis. Radon concentrations are measured in units of picocuries per liter of air, and 1 pCi/L is the average radon level chosen for the risk calculations (described later in this chapter). There are many houses with radon concentrations far above 1 pCi/L, particularly in Maine and Sweden. About 70 percent of the homes monitored in Maine had radon concentrations above 1 pCi/L. The houses in Sweden were preselected according to earlier geological surveys and

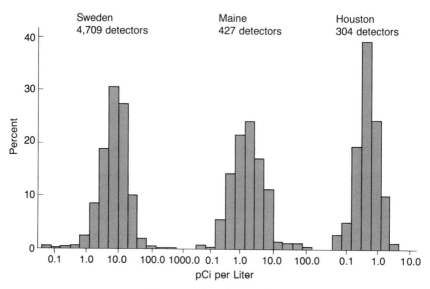

Fig. 3.2. Percentage of homes with indoor radon concentrations between values shown on the horizontal axis. Source: H. W. Alter, *Indoor Radon Levels: Field Experience Using the Track Etch® Method* (Walnut Creek, CA: Terradex Corporation, 1981). Reprinted by permission of the author.

particular construction practices that lead to high radon levels; Swedish homes in general have much less radon. Occupants of homes with these high radon-daughter concentrations may suffer exposures large enough to increase the risk of lung cancer during their lifetimes by a few percent or more.[5]

Many sites in the United States have relatively high levels of indoor radon and its daughters, owing to the presence of natural sources. But only a few studies have been performed, and the number of buildings involved is therefore not known. One study found a group of houses in a rural area of Maryland with significantly higher radon levels than the local average, which itself was high.[6] Locations in Maine, Illinois, Butte, Montana, and eastern Pennsylvania also have elevated radon levels in a significant fraction of houses studied. Of additional importance are sites contaminated through human activity. In Grand Junction, Colorado, a town of 20,000 people, it was discovered that several thousand houses were constructed on land where uranium mill tailings were used for fill. These tailings contain all of the radium originally present in the uranium ore; consequently, radon and radon daughters have been measured at very high levels in many buildings. A few hundred houses have been cleaned up at a cost of approximately $20,000 each. This continuing program should be completed in a few more years.

Phosphate rock is extensively mined in Florida, and the tailings from the strip mines are returned to the site and covered with the original soil. Large areas of this reclaimed land, which is high in radium content, have been sold for redevelopment, and thousands of houses built on it. Measurements in over a hundred units show high concentrations of radon daughters.[7]

Not only is the ground a source of radon; the building itself may unintentionally be made to emit radon. Phosphate wastes have been used in the manufacture of insulation installed in residences in the state of Washington, and in concrete used for foundations in Idaho. In Sweden, lightweight concrete containing alum shale was used for home construction until its radium content was found to cause high radon and radon-daughter concentrations in residential buildings.

The Health Effects of Radon Exposure

The main health hazard from exposure to radon and its daughters is an increased risk of lung cancer resulting from a radiation dose to lung tissue. The more significant risk is not from radon itself, but from two of the four short-lived daughters of radon that may be inhaled into the lungs, either directly or by attaching themselves to airborne particles. It is thought that most inhaled radon daughters are deposited in the bronchial region of the respiratory system. Since the first four radon daughters have short half-lives (30 minutes or less for each), as they decay they can expose the surrounding tissue to a great deal of radiation before being cleared from the lungs.

Two of the radon daughters decay by the emission of alpha particles (positively charged helium nuclei) and two decay by the emission of beta particles (electrons). The primary hazard is due to the alpha emissions of the two polonium isotopes. Since alpha particles have a shorter range than beta particles, more energy is deposited in a smaller section of tissue. Alpha particles have the potential to inflict 10 to 20 times the biological damage on tissue as electrons or x-rays of a similar energy. At the atomic level, energetic particles may separate electrons from their atoms, creating charged particles called ions. These ions also move through body tissue, creating further damage.

Considerable evidence has accumulated to indicate that the cell, and particularly its nucleus, is the primary site of radiation damage. Much more radiation is needed to kill a cell outright than to damage the nucleus. Damage to the nucleus can cause the cell to grow uncontrollably as a cancer cell. If enough cells become deranged, the tissue, then the organ itself, becomes disordered. A full-fledged case of lung cancer usually takes years to develop after the initial radiation damage. Radiation can also disrupt enough chemical bonds of a chromosome to break it into fragments, resulting in mutation.

Much of our knowledge about the human health effects of radon and its daughters comes from the experience of underground uranium miners. These miners were exposed to radiation from radon and its daughters at dose rates much higher than would ordinarily be experienced by occupants of residential buildings, and they developed lung cancer at a higher rate than the general population.

Epidemiological studies in several countries have shown an association between the incidence of lung cancer in uranium miners and cumulative exposure of radiation from radon decay products.[8] However, the cumulative exposures at which these cancer studies were made are generally higher by ten times or more than those characteristic of the normal indoor environment. Thus, in order to predict the health effects of indoor radon exposure, it is necessary to extrapolate beyond the range of exposures for which effects are definitely known.

As the cumulative radiation dose increases, so does the risk of getting lung cancer, but data are unavailable for low doses. To assess the effects of the low cumulative doses experienced by building occupants, it is necessary to make educated guesses. This problem is common to most research on the health effects of radiation, since most of the data on this subject come from studies of accidents, earlier medical use of radiation, and victims of military nuclear bombs, where high doses of radiation were involved.

There is an average latency period of approximately twenty years between exposure to radon and the onset of cancer among the miners. Almost all of the cancers in miners followed exposures of at least ten years. Those who smoked contracted cancer a few years sooner and slightly more often than nonsmokers.

In assessments of health effects at lower exposures, a commonly used assumption is that the incidence of lung cancer is always proportional to the cumulative dose from radon decay products. This assumption is known as the *linear hypothesis*; that is, it is assumed that there is no smallest or threshold dose for cancer induction and that doubling the radiation dose doubles the cancer incidence. Not all researchers agree with this assumption, but many do, and U.S. government publications on health risk analysis accept this hypothesis.

Data from epidemiological studies of uranium miners in this and other countries show that the number of lung cancers per unit of exposure to

Table 3.1. Representative Exposures
to Radon Daughters

Population or location	Exposure (WLM)
Uranium miners	100–1,000
Outdoors	<1.0
Indoors	10.0

SOURCE: National Research Council, *Indoor Pollutants* (Washington, DC: National Academy Press, 1981).

radon daughters range from 2.2 to 10 cases per million persons per year per working-level month (WLM) for the various studies.[9] The unit of radiation exposure, WLM, was devised for measuring the monthly exposure of mine workers to radon daughters. Using the linear hypothesis, the probable lung cancer risk to residential building occupants can be estimated.

Table 3.1 lists the cumulative exposure to radon daughters for uranium miners and the general population. For the general population, it is assumed that they spend 80 percent of their time indoors exposed to average levels of radon daughters. If we assume an incidence rate of 5 per million persons per WLM and a cumulative exposure of 10 WLM, then the total U.S. population of over 200 million people can expect about 10,000 cases of lung cancer per year from indoor radon exposure.

A large degree of uncertainty in this risk estimate is due to several factors. First, there is a wide range in the cancer incidence rates (from 2 to 10 cases per million persons per year per WLM) obtained for uranium miners in several epidemiological studies. Second, uranium miners differ from the general population. They have different breathing rates due to different activity levels, dissimilar age and sex distributions, and so forth. Third, the linear hypothesis may be wrong or only partly right.

If this estimate is correct, then approximately 10 percent of U.S. lung cancers are caused by indoor radon-daughter exposure. Since approximately 80 percent of all lung cancers (about 100,000 per year) are thought to be caused by cigarette smoking, this estimate would imply that most of the lung cancers occurring in nonsmokers are caused by radon-daughter exposure. Given all the uncertainties cited above, this is a highly controversial inference. A similar estimate, however, was independently arrived at for the Norwegian population by Dr. E. Stranden, of the Norwegian State Institute of Radiation Hygiene: "The exposure of the population from inhalation of radon daughters may account for about 10 percent of the total lung cancer incidence in the population."[10] Therefore, while the health risk from radon-daughter exposure is highly uncertain, the significant potential for harmful effects must be taken seriously.

Actually, it may be worse than this. Some researchers argue that part of the lung cancer attributed to smoking has exposure to radon daughters as a co-factor; that is, many lung cancers in smokers may be due to radiation from inhaling radon daughters coupled with damaged lung function from smoking.

The controversy over the effects of radiation in the indoor environment heated up when the Department of Energy proposed a program to weatherize millions of existing residential buildings in the United States. Weatherization includes reductions in infiltration rate through tightening of these houses. The EPA concluded that this energy conservation program could result in an additional 10,000 to 20,000 lung cancer deaths per year because of increased concentrations of radon and its decay products caused by reduced infiltration rates. Weatherization is discussed in Chapter 7.

Measurement and Control Techniques

An inexpensive radon measurement device is available from a California company; this track-etch alpha-particle detector provides a time-integrated measure of radon exposure, which is known to be highly variable. It is a passive device with no moving parts and requires no electric supply. The detector can be left in a suitable indoor location for periods of 3 months to a year and then sent back to the supplier for analysis. Appendix B contains more information about this company and another company that performs radon measurements.

If high indoor radon concentrations (greater than a few pCi/L) are found indoors, there are several things that can be done. Techniques for controlling indoor concentrations of radon and its daughters include measures that decrease the sources of radon, reduce transport of radon from its sources to the indoors, remove radon and its daughters from indoor air, and exchange inside air with outside air. The easiest method is to increase air exchange by opening windows or using fans. The tradeoff is in drafts and higher energy bills.

Building Materials and Site Selection

When new buildings are constructed, careful selection of building materials can be very effective in reducing that source of radon in the indoor environment. Systematic measurements of radon emanation rates from various building materials are being performed, allowing builders to choose low radon emitters for their project.

There is often less control over site election, but if construction must take place on land with high natural radioactivity, then special measures can be taken to reduce the transport of radon from the soil to the inside. In some situations, such as the phosphate lands in Florida, perhaps residential construction should be disallowed altogether. In Grand Junction, Colorado, soil with high radium content has been excavated from beneath houses and schools and replaced with soil of low radium content.

If well water is relatively high in radon content, as in parts of Maine, substituting surface water for domestic purposes will lower indoor radon concentrations.

Reducing the movement of radon from the soil to the indoor environment is a less costly approach than soil removal, but also less permanent. A method that was used successfully in Canadian rehabilitation programs is to seal cracks in basement walls and concrete slabs with polymeric caulks to keep radon-bearing air out. In some cases, epoxy paint and polyethylene films have been used as sealants. Though effective, these sealants must retain their integrity for long-term reduction of transport. Caulking and sealing may promote a buildup of radon and its daughters behind the barrier, causing an increase in gamma (long-range) radiation in the residence, but on the whole the effect is positive. The transport of radon indoors may also be reduced by ventilating crawlspaces or basements located beneath the living quarters.

Air Cleaning

Radon daughters (though not radon itself) may be removed from indoor air by collecting them or the particulates they are attached to. The effect of various air-cleaning methods on radon-daughter levels is complex and not fully understood. If more attached than unattached radon daughters are removed from the indoor air, the ratio of unattached to attached daughters will increase. According to some models of radiation dosage to the lungs from radon-daughter inhalation, this may increase the dose from radon daughters. The mechanisms by which air-cleaning devices function and their commercial availability are discussed in Chapter 8.

Heat Exchangers

Air-to-air heat exchangers, devices that are discussed in detail in Chapter 8, are effective in reducing radon and radon-daughter concentrations in residential buildings. The heat exchanger can remove contaminated indoor air and exchange it with outside air, while recovering much of the heat energy that might otherwise be lost from the indoor air. Thus, the ventilation rate may be increased in an energy-efficient manner. The Lawrence Berkeley Laboratory and other groups have been investigating

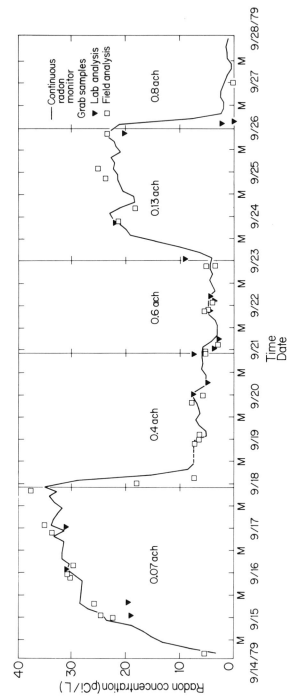

Fig. 3.3. Indoor radon concentration for a 2-week period in the National Association of Home Builders research house. The ventilation rate was changed by adjusting the airflow through a heat exchanger. ach, air changes per hour; M, midnight. Source: W. W. Nazaroff et al., *The Use of Mechanical Ventilation with Heat Recovery for Controlling Radon and Radon Daughter Concentrations in Houses,* Lawrence Berkeley Laboratory Report LBL-10222 (1980).

the performance of heat exchangers in laboratory and field tests. Figure 3.3 illustrates the ability of a heat exchanger to lower indoor radon concentrations in the National Association of Home Builders (NAHB) research house in Maryland.[11] Measurements over a 2-week period show that the radon concentration can be reduced from more than 30 pCi/L to 3 pCi/L when a heat exchanger is utilized.

Conclusion

Radon, a radioactive gas, is a naturally occurring indoor air pollutant. Building location is probably the major determinant of indoor radon and radon-daughter concentrations. Radon daughters that are inhaled may lodge in the upper reaches of the lungs for a long enough time period to deliver a large dose of radiation to the lungs. There is little doubt that increasing radon-daughter concentrations are associated with increasing human lung cancer incidence, but there is much debate over the magnitude of the risk in the general population from indoor exposure. Corrective action should probably be taken to lower radon and radon-daughter levels in homes with greater than a few picocuries per liter radon concentration. A number of effective radon control strategies are now available for use in existing residential buildings.

One method of determining which houses have high radon levels, short of performing measurements in 90 million households, would be to identify those areas of the United States with high radium concentrations in the soil. Such locations should then be chosen for further investigation, particularly radon measurements in some fraction of the homes in the geographic location. After this work is carried out, a much better estimate can be made of the potential health risk from exposure to radiation from radon and its daughters. Additionally, all houses in areas with high radon concentrations may be monitored, allowing for the application of control measures to reduce indoor radon levels.

4

Particulates

Everyone who has watched a sunbeam knows that the air is full of particles. They are not exactly constituents of the air like oxygen, and most are not exactly pollutants either. The fate of particles that reach the respiratory system depends on their size, shape, and density (see Fig. 4.1). Large particles are collected by the nasal sinuses and throat, and are eventually swallowed. Small particles penetrate farther into the respiratory system and may reach the alveoli. All of this is normal and usually harmless. A few classes of particulate matter are of more concern, especially if they remain trapped in the bronchial tubes or alveoli. The health effects caused by particulates range from a sneeze to lung cancer.

It stretches a point to call a single molecule a particle, but air ions, the first class of particulates to be discussed, can be that small or, when attached to something else, large enough to see. Other particulate pollutants to be discussed are asbestos, fiberglass, airborne microbes, and allergens. Particulates arising from combustion are discussed in Chapters 5 and 6. Treating particulate pollution involves source control and removal more than dilution. We will merely touch upon methods of treatment here; a detailed discussion follows in Chapter 8.

Air Ions

We are all aware of the ability of weather to change our moods. Certain hot dry winds such as the mistral in southern France, the Santa Ana in southern California, and the sharav in Israel are known to have physical and psychological effects in humans and animals. These winds have been blamed for causing headaches, nervousness, depression, and other

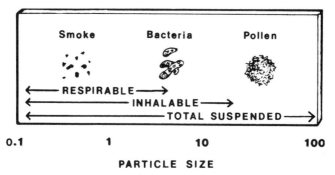

PARTICLE SIZE

Fig. 4.1. Sizes of airborne particles, in micrometers. Inhalable particles enter the respiratory tract. Respirable particles penetrate to the lungs. For size comparison, paper is about 100 micrometers thick. Source: *Indoor Air Quality Handbook* (Albuquerque, NM: Sandia National Laboratories and AnaChem, Inc., 1982).

ills. Some people think that the winds are even responsible for an increase in the rate of murders, suicides, and accidents. No wonder they are known as the witches' winds.

The connection between these winds and their effect on humans has proved elusive for thousands of years, but the solution may now be at hand. A number of scientists investigating these phenomena think that the winds produce changes in the electrical balance in the air and that this imbalance can affect our mental and physical well-being.

Nearly all gas molecules in the air are uncharged, that is, they have an equal number of protons (positive charges) and electrons (negative charges). There are a number of ways in which these molecules can become charged, each involving the addition of enough energy to an electron to free it from the pull of the positively charged nucleus. The loss of the electron leaves a positively charged molecule behind, a positive ion. The electron can be captured by a neutral molecule such as oxygen, creating a negative ion. Ions are created by lightning, cosmic rays, sunlight, radiation from radioactive materials, the movement of water droplets over waterfalls, and the rapid movement of great volumes of air over a land mass.

Small-sized air ions are found in very low concentrations in air; in clean mountain air there may be as many as one air ion for every 10^{15} molecules (or one in a million billion). They have a lifespan of minutes because they soon collide with other molecules in the air, becoming neutralized, or they become attached to neutral particles, producing large ions. The extremely low concentration of air ions might seem to rule out their participation in biological reactions; however, carefully controlled experiments have indicated that the biological effects of air ions must be taken seriously. Besides, the accepted limits of biological responsiveness have been extended by research showing that animals react to extremely small stimuli, for example, being able to see a few photons of light or smell a few molecules of odorant.

In the 1950's there was great interest in air ions. Devices that generated air ions were sold under claims of being able to cure anything from headaches to cancer. The Food and Drug Administration stopped these advertisements, and no medical claims are now allowed in extolling the virtues of air ion generators. Because of these misrepresentations, serious air ion research was greatly impeded for many years.

Fresh mountain or ocean air contains about equal numbers of small positive and negative ions (3,000 to 4,000 per cubic centimeter). Air inside buildings may have less than 100 ions per cubic centimeter. Since ions are neutralized by heating, ventilation, and cooling systems and by particulates in the air, there is a smaller number of air ions inside buildings. Some of the research performed to date indicates that an ion balance or an excess of negative ions may be beneficial to humans, and that air with an excess of positive ions or very few ions may be harmful.

Some of the first carefully controlled experiments on the biological effects of air ions were carried out in the 1950's by the late Albert Krueger, a professor of bacteriology at the University of California. Krueger found that the amount of serotonin in the blood and brains of mice was reduced by negative ions and raised by positive ions.[1] The result of an increase in serotonin (an allergy-producing hormone) is sleeplessness, irritability, stomach upset, and breathing difficulties.

These symptoms are similar to those observed in people exposed to hot dry winds. The sharav produces illness in about 30 percent of the exposed population. The illness, in the form of migraine headaches, nausea, vomiting, breathing difficulties, and irritability, was found to occur 24 to 28 hours before the strong winds, just when the total air ion count rose with a large positive-ion imbalance. Those falling ill from the sharav excrete abnormal amounts of serotonin in their urine. This suggests a connection between increasing positive-air-ion counts and increasing serotonin levels (and the adverse effects of serotonin) in the blood of exposed individuals. Some of the ions in the air we breathe are carried to the alveoli in our lungs, where they enter the bloodstream and are transported throughout our bodies. Positive ions cause the release of serotonin and negative ions inhibit it. Present theory holds that it is the serotonin that is largely responsible for the unpleasant symptoms.

Felix Sulman, of the Hebrew University of Jerusalem, has found that treatment with both serotonin-blocking drugs and negative ions provided relief in most victims of the sharav.[2] In 75 percent of cases, negative ions alone provided relief. In other studies, Sulman found that negative ions promoted alertness and relaxation in human subjects.

There have been numerous claims of benefits resulting from the use of negative-ion generators. Negative-ion therapy afforded complete relief to some migraine sufferers in clinical studies in England.[3] There have been reports of negative-ion therapy curing infant asthmatics.[4] Igho Kornblueh and associates at Northeastern Hospital in Philadelphia found that burn patients were helped by negative ions: their burns dried out and healed faster, with less scarring.[5] The patients exposed to negative ions experienced less pain and were more optimistic.

Sales of ion generators are growing rapidly, and companies manufacturing such devices are conducting aggressive advertising campaigns. Prices range from less than $100 for desktop units to thousands of dollars for large units that ionize the air in a large building. Advertisers claim that ion generators will remove cigarette smoke, pollen, pet dander, dust, odors, and other pollutants from the air. The generators are also claimed to reduce the levels of bacteria, mildew, and fungus spores. Besides enhancing the ion balance of rooms, ion generators play a part in other pollution control strategies. Thus, the mechanisms by which ion generators operate and how well they work will be discussed in Chapter 8, on general control techniques for indoor air pollutants.

Given the interest in and potential applications of ion technology, there are several steps that should be taken to determine the usefulness of negative-ion generators. First, an independent testing group, such as Consumers Union, should determine the ion production capabilities of such devices and their ability to remove particulates of various kinds from the air. Second, further well-controlled clinical tests of the biological effects of negative ions are necessary. Twenty to 30 percent of the population may benefit from the use of ion generators, but consumers have no simple way of determining whether they fall in this group. Until such tests are carried out, the use of negative-ion generators for their beneficial health effects will remain a controversial subject.

Asbestos

Asbestos is a name used for several magnesium silicate minerals that are fibrous in structure and resistant to damage by fire. Asbestos fibers are widely used because of their desirable thermal- and electric-insulating properties and their resistance to chemical degradation. Among the chief products made from asbestos are pipe covering, brake linings, plaster, plasterboard, and thermal and acoustic insulation. It is also used in roofing and flooring products, textiles, cement, and papers and felts. In the United States, over 70 percent of the asbestos produced each year is used in the construction business.

A once-common practice in the construction of high-rise office buildings was to spray fireproofing material containing from 10 to 30 percent asbestos onto girders and other structural components. Although the spraying of asbestos-containing materials ceased in 1978 after the Environmental Protection Agency banned it, the easily pulverizable material is still a significant source of indoor-generated asbestos. Children attending schools that contain asbestos on walls, ceilings, and other exposed surfaces are a population of great concern. These materials can be damaged during routine activities and by purposeful destructive behavior. The state of California has provided $45 million to remove asbestos from its public schools. A survey has shown that 3,200 of the 7,000 school buildings contain easily crumbled asbestos.

In the twenty-story San Francisco Federal Building, it has been determined that asbestos was being circulated through the air-conditioning system that serves 4,300 government workers. The problem originates in crawlspaces above offices where asbestos fireproofing sprayed on structural beams and on the floors above is crumbling because of age and construction damage. Some of the asbestos dust is carried by the air delivery system to the offices below. Although the asbestos levels found within the building are below the Occupational Safety and Health Administration standard of 2 fibers per cubic centimeter, a potential health hazard still exists for building occupants, according to a National Bureau of Standards draft report.[6] The national bureau is conducting studies of the asbestos hazard in eight other major federal buildings. In fact, OSHA recently proposed a lowering of the asbestos standard to one-half fiber per cubic centimeter.

Through occupational health studies it has been determined that people who work with asbestos have a higher risk of developing lung cancer, mesothelioma, and certain gastrointestinal cancers. Mesothelioma is a cancer, ordinarily extremely rare, that develops on the mesothelium or lining of the chest cavity. Asbestosis is an irreversible and disabling lung disease resulting from the retention of inhaled asbestos particles in the lung. Asbestos insulation workers have a significantly higher incidence of lung cancer and mesothelioma than control groups similar in all other ways except for exposure to asbestos. Smokers exposed to asbestos are much more likely to die from lung cancer than exposed nonsmokers. These cancers often take 20 to 30 years to develop and may sometimes come from short-term (less than a year) exposures to asbestos. Spouses and children of asbestos workers also appear to be at higher risk of contracting mesothelioma and lung cancer, thanks to asbestos brought home on the workers' clothing. The threshold for cancer induction by asbestos fibers is unknown.

A great deal of asbestos is still present in many homes.[7] Do-it-yourselfers using old spackling compound to tape joints on wallboard can be exposed to asbestos because at one time most spackle contained 12 to 15 percent asbestos. Some papier-mâché used until recently by the New York City Board of Education contained approximately 50 percent asbestos; the Board disposed of 50,000 five-pound bags of this material intended for kindergarten use. There may still be asbestos textiles in the home, such as asbestos gloves, or do-it-yourself carpenters may have old asbestos cement board. Even clothing can sometimes contain asbestos fibers.

Thousands of homes and apartments built in the 1940's and 1950's contain furnaces and air ducts insulated with asbestos.[8] As furnaces age, invisible asbestos fibers may be released into the ventilation system of the home. Nowadays the insulation of choice is fiberglass. A contractor who has removed asbestos from Los Angeles schools estimates the cost of removing or encapsulating a typical residential heating system at between $500 and $1,200. Many experts on the health risks of asbestos say that any crumbling asbestos insulation found in a home should be professionally removed or coated.

The U.S. Consumer Product Safety Commission has banned the use of asbestos textiles in general-use garments, asbestos in artificial fireplace materials, and asbestos-containing spackling and taping compounds. Voluntary actions by manufacturers controlled the use of asbestos in hand-held hair dryers. Where asbestos-containing materials are identified in existing buildings, a number of strategies are possible. Material that is in good condition and difficult to reach can be covered and left undisturbed. A false ceiling will help but is usually not practicable in a house. When repairs or remodeling is done, additional precautions must be taken. Asbestos-containing material that is easily pulverized may have to be removed entirely.

Fiberglass

A few words should be said about fiberglass insulation. Both rock wool and glass wool are fibrous glasses. Since the fibers in the glass wool used for home insulation can be similar in size and shape to asbestos fibers, it is prudent to ask if glass fibers have effects similar to those of asbestos fibers. Indeed, lung tumors have been induced in animals by implanting glass fibers, and some studies of the cancer induction process associated with fibers indicate that a fiber's dimensions are more important than its chemistry.

Nevertheless, a recent 4-year study by Los Alamos National Laboratory found no ill effects in rats and hamsters forced to breathe fiberglass fibers.[9] The study was part of an ongoing 7-year effort funded by the Thermal Insulation Manufacturers Association. There was no indication of inflammatory diseases, such as pneumonia, or chronic diseases that cause changes in the lung, such as fibrosis or pneumoconiosis, in the animals autopsied. The researchers will concentrate next on animal studies using actual fibers from fiberglass insulating materials.

Fibrous glass materials can indeed produce severe skin irritation in people working with them (a problem prevented by wearing long sleeves and gloves) and can also be irritating to the eyes and, if inhaled, the upper respiratory tract. But no epidemiological study has demonstrated substantial health hazards related to fibrous materials other than asbestos that may contaminate the indoor environment. It seems prudent to minimize exposure to small glass fibers if only to avoid irritation. More serious health problems might also be averted, but there is as yet no scientific evidence of that.

Airborne Microbes and Allergens

Large airborne particles usually trigger nothing more serious than blinking or perhaps a sneeze, but smaller-sized particulates may have profound medical effects. We will address here two classes of particulates: microbes and allergens. The first group has undergone intensive study in public dwellings, such as hotels, in connection with infrequent but newsworthy outbreaks of disease. The second is well known in most households, where the effects are humbler and more frequent, but has received less scientific scrutiny.

Viruses and Bacteria

Most airborne viruses and bacteria are generated indoors by building occupants themselves. They are most often exhaled from the respiratory tract by breathing, coughing, or sneezing, but may also be shed in feces or urine and from wounds on the skin. Humidifiers, which have a reservoir of heated water, can incubate microbes that enter the air. There are cases, too, where outdoor sources of airborne microbes have caused infection indoors. For example, in the San Francisco Bay Area, Q fever was disseminated from a tannery to residents of houses and apartments downwind.[10]

Infectious particles released indoors, like ordinary dust particles, remain airborne for periods ranging from seconds to hours. Larger particles usually infect people who are close to the source, since they tend to settle out before traveling far; smaller particles may infect people some distance away.

Airborne viruses and bacteria may cause influenza, pneumonia, and other diseases and are the most important cause of acute respiratory illness in the United States. These illnesses lead to millions of lost days of work and billions of dollars in lost production every year. Although these illnesses are also spread by contact with sick people, airborne infection can be the dominant mode of transfer, depending on the particular microbe. Some well-known airborne microbes include the measles virus, Asian influenza virus, tuberculosis bacilli, and *Legionella*. The common cold is spread primarily by touch.

There are numerous examples of airborne microbes being dispersed through a school or office building and infecting people who had no physical contact with the source of contagion. Epidemiologist R. C. Riley studied an epidemic of measles in an elementary school near Rochester that began with a second-grade girl.[11] Twenty-eight secondary cases followed, after an incubation period of about 10 days, in fourteen classrooms served by the same ventilation system. In most nonresidential buildings, mechanical ventilation systems are used to supply outside air to the occupants via a system of fans and ductwork. In this school's ventilation system, as in many others, air is recirculated from one room to another before it is exhausted to the outside. Since the first girl to be infected with measles did not occupy the same room as the other children who became infected, Riley concluded that the measles virus reached its victims through the ventilation system.

Influenza virus is thought to be transmitted by the airborne route. Epidemics of influenza in the United States and other countries have caused many thousands of deaths and millions of illnesses. In this country an average of more than 10,000 deaths from influenza occur each year.[12]

A number of factors have helped to reduce the aerial transfer of disease. Less crowded living conditions, isolation of infected persons, and vaccination of large portions of the population are some of the more important ones. Other control techniques, such as the use of high-efficiency air filters, will be discussed in Chapter 8.

Allergenic Agents

Housedust and plant pollens are two of the most important factors in provoking symptoms of allergic rhinitis (hay fever) and asthma. Rhinitis affects about 15 percent of the population, and asthma affects about 3 to 5 percent. Allergy to animal dander is also very common.

Allergic individuals are predisposed to secrete large amounts of an antibody when exposed to an allergen they are sensitive to. When an antigen-antibody reaction takes place, histamine and other substances are released. Allergic reactions can take place anywhere on the skin or in the nose, airways, and alveoli. The effects on the particular body tissue involved include the dilation of blood vessels, mucous secretion, contraction of the bronchial smooth muscles, and cellular inflammation. The symptoms are stuffy or runny noses in the case of allergic rhinitis and difficulty in breathing in the case of asthma. Severe allergic reactions may send the victim to the hospital.

Much has been written on allergenic agents. Some of the more important air allergens in the indoor environment will be briefly discussed below.

Many different pollens from grass, trees, and flowers have been shown to cause allergic rhinitis and asthma. Pollen counts vary greatly by geographical location and season and are also generally greater outdoors than indoors. Pollen grains are generally too large to penetrate beyond the trachea in the respiratory system, although fragments of pollen grains sometimes reach the lower airways.

Housedust is an important cause of allergic rhinitis and asthma in climates where winters are humid and mild, such as along the west coast of the United States and Europe and in parts of Japan. In these climates, the main source of the antigen is housedust mites. These barely visible organisms, which feed on human skin scales, feathers, and fungi, are too big to become airborne and be inhaled. The airborne allergen probably arises from the mite's excreta, the particles of which are of an inhalable size. Mites are readily found in beds, mattresses, and pillows; they require high humidity (45 percent or more) and usually die in centrally heated homes when the heating season starts and indoor humidity drops. Many bacteria and molds also occur in housedust, but their contribution to the allergenic properties of housedust is not known. Roach fecal pellets are an important source of allergens, especially in homes with poor sanitary conditions.

Domestic animals, especially cats, are important causes of allergic rhinitis and asthma. The source of the allergen is dander, small scales from feathers or hair. The feces of birds, particularly those of pigeons and parakeets, contain allergens that cause allergic rhinitis and asthma, as well as a more serious disease, hypersensitivity pneumonitis. The occurrence of this disease in air-conditioned buildings will be discussed in Chapter 9, on indoor air quality problems in offices.

When buildings are made more energy-efficient by reducing ventilation, we need to consider the effect of this reduced air flow on the concentration of airborne allergens and microbes. Reduced infiltration may lead to longer retention of indoor-generated water vapor (from cooking, showering, etc.) and thus higher relative humidity. This tends to create a favorable environment for housedust mites, molds, and fungi. The problem is discussed further in Chapter 7.

A number of researchers believe that there is a relationship between respiratory illness and indoor relative humidity. More colds occur in the winter than in the summer, and during the winter the indoor relative humidity in heated buildings is relatively low compared to summer time. George Green, of the University of Saskatchewan, studied this relationship and found that "adding humidity to the air shows evidence of reducing absenteeism in adults and of a significant reduction in colds and/or absenteeism in children."[13] A humidifier can be used to add water vapor to the air. Electrical energy is required to heat a reservoir of water and cause some evaporation. Maintenance is needed to see that humidifiers do not incubate microorganisms. The water temperature is an important factor in determining how microorganisms grow in this water environment. The potential spread of allergies or disease from microorganisms that may grow in humidifiers is discussed in Chapter 9.

The suspected connection between respiratory illness and relative humidity derives from the study of ciliary movements. The cilia are the microscopic hairs in the conducting division of the respiratory tract that move the mucus and help clear the respiratory system of foreign particles. Mucous flow has been found to decrease with decreasing relative humidity by some researchers,[14] though not by all.[15] Another factor that may affect the contact transfer of colds is the survival rate of various organisms. The survival rate can increase or decrease with decreasing relative humidity, depending upon the particular virus. The effect of relative humidity on respiratory illness bears further study. The benefits of increased humidity need to be weighed against the costs (for example, increased energy use and possible increased growth of some allergenic microorganisms).

5

Combustion Products

There are numerous possible sources of combustion products in a residence: cooking appliances, space heaters, furnaces, fireplaces, and cigarettes. Factors that influence the indoor concentration of air contaminants resulting from combustion include the nature of the fuel, the location of the source, the quantity of air used, the temperature of combustion, and the presence or absence of a ventilation system.

Characteristics of Combustion Products

Smoke is the first product of combustion that may come to mind, but smokeless burning likewise releases combustion products. Because it often smells and is visible, smoke is easily detected and is usually treated promptly. (Tobacco smoke, the subject of Chapter 6, is the exception.) The "clean-burning" combustion sources—stoves, space heaters, and such—have health effects that are also significant in the indoor environment. The most potent ingredients of combustion-related pollution do not smell strongly and are invisible.

Carbon monoxide is a colorless, odorless, toxic gas that is produced by the incomplete burning of fuels containing carbon. An inadequate supply of air for combustion, such as occurs in "airtight" wood-burning stoves and improperly maintained gas stoves and gas and oil furnaces, greatly increases the rate of carbon monoxide emission. If set wrong, flues and dampers restrict the flow of carbon monoxide and other combustion products to the outside, causing a buildup indoors.

Carbon monoxide measurements in a number of cities in the United States indicate that outdoor levels range from as little as 1 ppm to greater than 140 ppm for brief periods in heavy traffic. Commuters are often ex-

Table 5.1. Health Effects of Various Combustion Products

Contaminant	Health effect
Aldehydes	Irritation of eyes, nose, and throat
Carbon monoxide	Headaches, impairment of visual acuity and brain functioning; irregular heart functioning
Carbon dioxide	Headaches, dizziness, shortness of breath, and drowsiness
Nitric oxide	At high concentrations, irritation of eyes, nose, and throat
Nitrogen dioxide	Damage to lung tissue and increased airway resistance
Particulates	Varies according to chemical and physical properties; for example, benzo-*a*-pyrene is carcinogenic, other particulates may or may not have adverse health effects
Sulfur dioxide	Irritation of skin, eyes, and mucous membranes; at high concentration, constriction of upper airways

N O T E : See the appropriate sections of the text for information on the exposures necessary to cause the health effects listed.

posed to concentrations of 50 ppm or more. Measurements by the Environmental Protection Agency in more than 100 vehicles (buses, taxis, police cars) indicated that in 58 percent of the 120 personal sampler readings for rides longer than 8 hours, the EPA 8-hour air quality standard for carbon monoxide (9 ppm) was exceeded.[1]

Carbon monoxide interferes with the body's oxygen transport by binding to hemoglobin more strongly than oxygen does. The resulting carboxyhemoglobin cannot carry oxygen to the body's cells. The symptoms of carbon monoxide poisoning are dizziness, blurred vision, and rapid breathing (see Table 5.1). At very high concentrations of carbon monoxide (1,500 ppm for 1 hour), death may result. Adverse physiological effects begin at a carboxyhemoglobin level of about 2.5 percent; exposure to air with 50 ppm carbon monoxide for 90 minutes, or 15 ppm for 10 hours, is enough to reach this level, at which time interval discrimination is impaired. Such exposures are possible in heavy traffic. Carboxyhemoglobin levels above 5 percent have produced evidence of physiologic stress in patients with heart disease.[2] The current EPA standard for carbon monoxide is mainly justified on the basis of preventing adverse effects in patients with cardiac and peripheral vascular disease.

Carbon dioxide is not normally thought of as a pollutant; however, at high concentrations it may cause headaches, loss of judgment, and asphyxiation. It is a colorless, odorless gas that is formed whenever carbon-containing substances are burned. Typical outdoor concentrations range from 300 to 330 ppm. Studies of submarine personnel have shown that there are some slight respiratory effects from exposure to between 10,000 and 30,000 ppm of carbon dioxide. The occupational health standard is 5,000 ppm.

At high temperatures, nitrogen and oxygen in the air react to form *nitrogen oxides* (nitrogen dioxide and nitric oxide). These temperatures are produced when natural gas and kerosene are burned; wood fires are not strong sources. The deleterious health effects of nitrogen oxides (increased upper respiratory infections) are generally attributable to nitrogen dioxide, a toxic gas that is a respiratory irritant. However, nitric oxide may also be harmful, since it binds to hemoglobin to produce methemoglobin, and many of the adverse health effects attributed to carbon monoxide may result from the presence of nitric oxide as well.

At concentrations of 0.05 ppm, typical in homes with gas cooking or unvented space heaters, nitrogen dioxide may affect sensory perception, especially adaptation to darkness, and may produce eye irritation. A number of studies have shown that short-term exposure to nitrogen dioxide at a concentration between 1.0 and 3.0 ppm for less than 1 hour increases airway resistance in humans.[3]

The combustion of kerosene and natural gas gives rise to a number of organic compounds including formaldehyde, whose health effects are discussed in Chapter 2. Wood-burning stoves are also a source of formaldehyde and various gaseous pollutants.

Particulates

Most of the particulates in smoke result from the incomplete combustion of burning materials such as tobacco and wood. A smoldering cigarette or smoky wood fire may release large quantities of small particulates.

The health effects arising from inhaling these particles depend strongly upon their chemical and physical nature. The size and density of a particle determine the probability of its reaching the lungs if inhaled. Its chemical nature determines the effect on lung tissue, if any. Benzo-*a*-pyrene, an organic particulate, is a carcinogenic compound produced during combustion of wood or animal dung. The particle may also interfere with one or more of the clearance mechanisms in the respiratory system. Particles larger than 15 micrometers are filtered out by the nose. Smaller inhalable particles can be deposited along the respiratory tract. Respirable particles, some as large as 10 micrometers, penetrate to the lungs, where they may be deposited or absorbed in the bloodstream and transported to other parts of the body. Particles deposited in the nose and windpipe are dislodged and exhaled or swallowed and excreted within several days. Particles deposited in the lungs have a greater potential for harm because of their longer period of contact with lung tissue.

Gas Stoves

Approximately 60 percent of U.S. homes use gas stoves for cooking. Studies that have monitored the concentration of various pollutants in residential buildings with gas stoves have almost all documented elevated levels of carbon monoxide and nitrogen oxides indoors. In some cases, concentrations exceeded the outdoor health standards. Other pollutants released from gas stoves during cooking are formaldehyde and respirable particulates.

Before discussing some specifics of the pollution related to cooking with gas, another aspect of gas stoves is worth mentioning. A study published in 1981 concluded, from an analysis of gas consumption in New York City dwellings, that about half of 340,000 households surveyed used their gas ranges for supplemental heat.[4] Whatever hazards arise from ordinary cooking must be magnified considerably for these households.

The nature and amount of pollutants emitted by gas stoves depend on the nature of the food being cooked, the frequency and duration of cooking, and the efficiency of combustion. Efficient combustion requires the right mixture of natural gas and air to be fed to the flame. A poorly tuned stove can emit much more carbon monoxide than a well-tuned stove. Emissions tend to be intermittent; pollutants reach peak concentration in the kitchen during times meals are prepared. These pollutants disperse throughout the house, and usually within an hour's time the concentration of pollutants is the same in the kitchen, bedrooms, and living room.

Numerous tests of gas stove emissions have been performed by researchers at the Lawrence Berkeley Laboratory in California. The results of one such test are shown below.[5] Figure 5.1 illustrates how carbon monoxide concentration varies during and after gas stove use in a 1,150-square-foot research house. During these tests, the oven was set at 350°F and the two top burners were set on high flame. A water-filled pot was placed on each burner, and oven and burners were operated for 35 minutes. The stove was new and was installed by a commercial service man without any special tuning procedure. This house had been tightened and thus had a low average infiltration rate of about 0.30 air changes per hour. The peak concentration of carbon monoxide in the kitchen (24 ppm) was much higher than outside (1 ppm), but still lower than the 1-hour outdoor air quality standard of 35 ppm. Almost 3 hours later, the con-

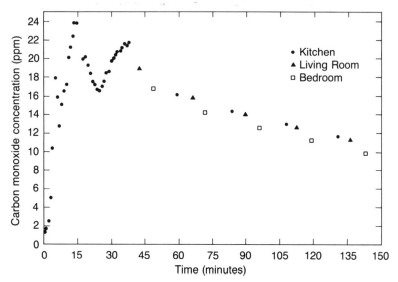

Fig. 5.1. Carbon monoxide concentrations in a house with the oven and two top burners on for 35 minutes. No exhaust fan was used. Source: G. W. Traynor *et al.*, *The Effects of Ventilation on Residential Air Pollution Due to Emissions from a Gas-Fired Range*, Lawrence Berkeley Laboratory Report LBL-12563 (1981).

centration throughout the house was 10 ppm. It is difficult to determine the health effects, if any, from such exposures without also measuring the carboxyhemoglobin level in the blood. The maximum allowable 8-hour average outdoor concentration is 9 ppm.

Two Canadian researchers have performed experiments indicating that the carbon monoxide concentration is highly dependent on the number of burners in operation and on whether or not the burners are covered with pans.[6] Figure 5.2 illustrates the buildup of carbon monoxide when one to four gas burners are in operation for 30 minutes. In the nine typical Canadian homes monitored in this study, the level of carbon monoxide after 20 minutes of stove operation ranged from 35 to 120 ppm. A possible reason for the higher levels in the Canadian study is that the stoves were not new and may have been less well tuned than those in the California study. The air exchange rates were not given for these homes, but the researchers stated that they were not specifically constructed to reduce air infiltration. Mechanical ventilation was not used while the stoves were in operation. Thus, both U.S. and Canadian studies show that carbon monoxide concentrations in homes with unvented gas stoves may exceed applicable health standards.

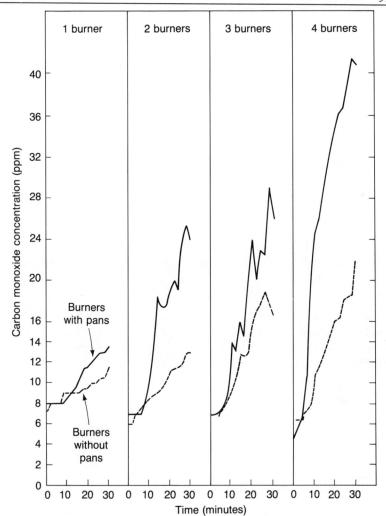

Fig. 5.2. Increases in carbon monoxide concentration when using one to four covered and uncovered burners. Source: T. D. Sterling and E. Sterling, "Carbon Monoxide Levels in Kitchens and Homes with Gas Cookers," *Air Pollution Control Association Journal*, vol. 29, no. 3 (March 1979). Reprinted by permission of the association.

Another important pollutant produced by gas stoves is nitrogen dioxide. Testing at a California research house with typical gas stove operation indicated that the concentration of nitrogen dioxide exceeded the California outdoor air quality standard of 0.25 ppm for a 1-hour exposure.[7] Peak 1-hour concentrations were greater than 0.40 ppm in both the kitchen and living room and just under 0.25 ppm in the bedroom. The infiltration rate varied between 0.33 and 0.44 air changes per hour during the course of this study.

The pollutant concentrations are significant, but another perspective reminds us that the gas range is far cleaner than older ways of cooking. Consider the stoves used in India, where wood and dung are the primary fuels. The East-West Center in Honolulu documented *average* particulate levels of 7,000 micrograms per cubic meter in Indian kitchens, or 27 times the U.S. 24-hour standard, and calculated an exposure to benzo-*a*-pyrene equivalent to smoking twenty packs of cigarettes a day.[8] India's National Institute of Occupational Health recorded extremely high concentrations of benzo-*a*-pyrene (up to 9.3 micrograms per cubic meter) and levels of average total suspended particulates of up to 26,000 micrograms per cubic meter—100 times the U.S. 24-hour standard.[9]

Researchers have sought to quantify the health effects of gas cooking through epidemiological studies. The results are not unambiguous.

Health Effects of Gas Cooking

Surveys in England and the United States have shown slightly higher rates of minor respiratory ailments and slightly impaired lung function in people living in homes where gas rather than electricity is used for cooking. At an international conference on indoor air pollution one paper, "The Case for Entirely Removing the Gas Range from Indoors," provoked a vigorous response from some gas industry representatives.[10] One gas utility representative cited studies by the Environmental Protection Agency of 146 homes on Long Island in New York and 441 homes in the suburbs of Columbus, Ohio, showing no significant difference in respiratory illnesses between those using gas and those using electricity in their homes. These epidemiological studies will be discussed in some detail to gain a better understanding of these conflicting findings.

In England, R. J. Melia, C. du V. Florey, and S. Chinn examined the lung health of 4,800 English and Scottish children aged 5 to 10.[11] The prevalence of respiratory symptoms or diseases was higher in children from homes where gas was used for cooking than in children from homes where electricity was used. The association appeared to be independent of age, sex, social class, and number of cigarette smokers in the household (though it appeared only in urban areas). The researchers found, for example, that boys living in homes with gas cooking have an 18 percent greater prevalence rate of respiratory illnesses than boys living in homes with electric cooking. The probability of this association being a chance result was only 1 percent.

For a sample of 103 boys and girls living in houses with gas stoves from the above study, nitrogen dioxide measurements were taken both indoors and outdoors. It was found that the prevalence of respiratory illness increased with increasing levels of nitrogen dioxide in the bedroom—not the kitchen. The mean bedroom concentration of nitrogen dioxide in the gas-cooking homes was twice that in the electric-cooking homes.

Frank Speizer of Harvard and his associates studied approximately 8,000 children from 6 to 10 years of age from six U.S. communities. Questionnaires were completed by their parents and simple lung function tests were performed in school.[12] Comparing children living in homes with gas stoves and those living in homes with electric stoves, Speizer found that children from gas households had a more extensive history of respiratory illness before age 2. Measurements taken in representative homes for 24-hour periods showed that nitrogen dioxide levels were two to three times higher in homes with gas stoves than in homes with electric stoves.

Lung function measurements were made using a spirometer, which records the quantity of air exhaled by a person as a function of time (see Fig. 5.3). The total volume of air exhaled (forced vital capacity , or FVC) and the forced expiratory volume in one second (FEV-1) were read from

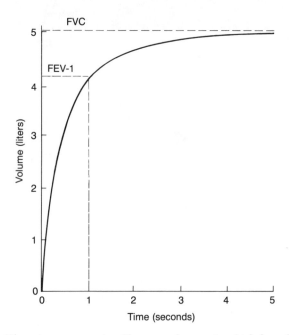

Fig. 5.3. The spirometer tracing illustrates the way in which forced vital capacity (FVC) and forced expiratory volume in 1 second (FEV-1) are calculated.

each tracing. It was found that children from homes with gas cooking had significantly lower FEV-1 and FVC than children from homes with electric cooking. Speizer and associates stated that they were using FVC as a crude indicator of lung size, recognizing that it did not include the residual volume of the lungs. They concluded, "We do not know whether the failure to reach full adult lung size is related to the subsequent susceptibility of developing obstructive lung disease, but it is not an untenable hypothesis that those persons with minor impairment of total lung growth are more susceptible to rapid decline in pulmonary function in adult life."

Two other studies reported an association between reduced forced expiratory volume (FEV) and the presence of a gas stove in the home. In the first study, in which the EPA surveyed over 16,000 school-aged children living in seven U.S. cities, a small decrease in forced expiratory volume in the first three-fourths of a second (FEV-0.75) was reported among girls 9 to 13 years old.[13] In a Johns Hopkins University study of 560 white males, there were almost three times as many adults with impaired ventilatory function (FEV-0.75 less than 80 percent of predicted value for age and size) in houses using gas as a cooking fuel as in houses cooking with electricity.[14]

Two other studies found no association between the use of gas stoves for cooking and either respiratory illness or pulmonary function. A 1-year study of 441 families living in the suburbs of Columbus, Ohio, found that although there was twice the average nitrogen dioxide concentration (0.05 ppm compared to 0.02 ppm for a 24-hour average) in homes with gas cooking as compared to homes with electric cooking, there was no increased incidence of respiratory illness among the 1,900 inhabitants.[15] Lung function tests (FVC and FEV-0.75) among 822 of the subjects showed no statistically significant difference between those living in houses with gas cooking and those living in houses with electric cooking.

The second study was conducted by the EPA in a suburban community in Long Island, New York.[16] It was found that the respiratory illness rates of mothers in gas- and electric-cooking households showed no statistically significant difference. Only 146 people took part in this study, and nitrogen dioxide measurements were not taken.

In summary, it appears that there may be some increase in respiratory illness and a small decrease in lung function among young children living in homes with gas cooking compared to those living in homes with electric cooking. The failure of the last two studies mentioned to confirm these results may be due to both the small number of total subjects and the small number of children surveyed. In addition, as will be discussed in the next chapter, there may be more-sensitive indicators of respiratory

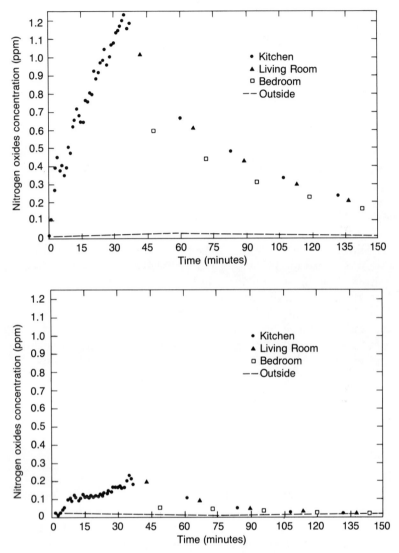

Fig. 5.4. Nitrogen oxides concentrations in a house with the oven and two top burners on for 35 minutes. The upper case is where a whole-house fan provides 0.83 air changes per hour of mechanical ventilation. In the lower case, an exhaust fan provides 1.5 ach of local ventilation. Source: G. W. Traynor *et al.*, *The Effects of Ventilation on Residential Air Pollution Due to Emissions from a Gas-Fired Range*, Lawrence Berkeley Laboratory Report LBL-12563 (1981).

impairment than forced expiratory volume. More studies utilizing better indicators may help clarify the question whether the use of gas stoves is associated with adverse respiratory health effects. Furthermore, there is no clear association between average nitrogen dioxide concentration and increased respiratory illness or decreased lung function in any of these studies. Another combustion product, or several acting together, may be responsible for the adverse health effects seen by some researchers.

Control of Gas Stove Emissions

Nitrogen dioxide and carbon monoxide concentrations can both be substantially reduced by the use of a range hood, a device over the stove consisting of a fan and associated ductwork that exhausts combustion products to the outdoors. Figure 5.4 illustrates the range hood's effectiveness in lowering nitrogen dioxide concentrations in several rooms of the California research house.[17] The top graph shows levels when a gas stove is operated for 35 minutes and a whole-house fan provides 0.83 air changes per hour of ventilation. In the lower figure, a range hood provides 1.5 ach of local ventilation. This is equivalent to an air flow of about 200 cubic feet per minute, easily obtainable from a small house fan. With the range hood, the peak concentration in the kitchen falls from 1.2 ppm to about 0.25 ppm. Local ventilation while a stove is in use is an effective measure for controlling all indoor air pollutants at the source. In cold weather the heating load increases when the range hood is used, because cold outside air replaces the warm inside air that is exhausted by the fan. However, the fan is used only intermittently, and the cost of heating the excess cold air is offset by the benefit of improved air quality.

Space Heating

Approximately 60 percent of U.S. homes burn natural gas as their primary heating fuel. In most of these homes, externally vented central furnaces are the appliance of choice. When these heating systems are properly designed and maintained, combustion products do not enter the indoor environment. However, if there is a faulty exhaust system (for example, a blocked flue) or if there is lower air pressure inside the building than outside, there can be emission of combustion products to the indoor space.

Kerosene Heaters

Until recent years, kerosene heaters were most prevalent in rural areas with mild winters, such as the southern United States. This type of space-heating appliance is more hazardous than externally vented systems because the combustion products are emitted directly into the room.

There are now more than twenty brands of portable kerosene heaters for sale by a dozen competitors.[18] More than ten million kerosene heaters are being used throughout the United States. The new kerosene heater is quite different from the ones that warmed homes during the Depression. Developed by the fuel-short Japanese, most of the heaters now have battery-powered electric ignition and a low center of gravity so they do not tip over easily. The stainless steel burner mechanism that controls the ratio of fuel to air works very well if adjusted properly; the kerosene burns with almost perfect efficiency and with little odor.

The high combustion efficiency is one of the factors allowing such heaters to provide low-cost heating and also keeps the output of carbon monoxide at a very low level. The kerosene heater can be used only where it is needed, and the heat is not lost up the chimney.

Several studies have been performed to assess the level of air contamination from these unvented space heaters. One was carried out in a test chamber at the Lawrence Berkeley Laboratory.[19] The test chamber was 900 cubic feet in volume, approximately the size of a kitchen or small bedroom. All kerosene heaters, two convective and two radiant, were found to emit carbon monoxide, nitrogen oxides, and formaldehyde, as well as the expected carbon dioxide. Convective heaters draw in cold air, pass it by the heat source, and discharge warm air. Radiant heaters radiate heat energy directly from the heat source, often assisted by reflectors. With both types of heater, carbon dioxide levels reached 10,000 ppm, twice the 8-hour occupational health standard, after an hour of operation. Nitrogen dioxide concentrations exceeded the California 1-hour standard of 0.25 ppm, by a factor of 7 for the convective heater and a factor of 2 for the radiant model. For radiant heaters, carbon monoxide concentrations were 1.4 times the 8-hour EPA standard of 9 ppm. It was found that adjusting the wick length improperly (contrary to the manufacturer's instructions) could increase the carbon monoxide emission rate by 8 times. During these experiments the heaters were operated for 1 hour, producing approximately 8,000 BTU of heat per hour (enough for a typical room in a cold climate), and the air exchange rate was 0.4 ach.

Pollutant emissions from kerosene heaters were also measured by scientists from Yale University.[20] They found that convective and radiant kerosene heaters "can result in concentrations of sulfur dioxide and nitrogen dioxide in excess of the relevant ambient air quality standards," and that carbon dioxide levels can exceed the standard of the Occupational Health and Safety Administration. They also determined that carbon monoxide concentrations could be of concern when a radiant heater is used in a small room with a moderate ventilation rate. Except for the sulfur dioxide finding (probably due to differences in kerosene fuel), there is good agreement between the results from these two laboratories.

Kerosene heaters are banned in several states, including Washington, Oregon, and Colorado. In California, retailers of unvented kerosene heaters must state, in their advertisements, that the heaters are not for residential use. It is well known, however, that most people buying the heaters intend to use them in their homes.

The Consumer Product Safety Commission held hearings on kerosene heaters in late 1982. Peter Preuss, head of the agency's health science division, said research by independent laboratories indicated that kerosene heaters exhausted two contaminants, nitrogen dioxide and sulfur dioxide, at a rate that had "a potential for exceeding the EPA's outdoor standards by a significant amount."[21] In 1983, the commission decided that instead of issuing mandatory standards, the government should continue to work with the manufacturers to improve voluntary standards and to develop new ones. The commission staff said that kerosene heaters used in a room fully open to the rest of the house are not likely to cause health problems for most people; "certain asthmatics and people with chronic lung diseases, however, may experience mild breathing difficulties," it said, especially if the heater is in a closed room. It appears that kerosene heaters should be used only in well-ventilated areas or in large rooms in order to lower the concentration of emitted pollutants. The heaters should not be used for long periods. For those who have not already bought a kerosene heater, it would be prudent to buy a vented model if it is to be used indoors.

Gas Space Heaters

Emissions from gas-fired space heaters are highly dependent on the size of the heater, the manufacturer, and the state of tuning of the appliance. Eight heaters, ranging in heat production from 12,000 to 40,000 BTU per hour, were tested in the same Lawrence Berkeley Laboratory chamber described above.[22] Nitrogen oxide and formaldehyde emission rates were found to be lower than for gas-fired stoves. However, the fuel consumption rate is generally greater for gas space heaters than for gas stoves, making them a more important source of indoor pollutants where they are used. Carbon monoxide and formaldehyde emission rates were found to be much more variable than those of other pollutants and very sensitive to the state of tuning for some heaters. After 30 minutes of operation, typical pollutant concentrations were 4,000 ppm of carbon dioxide, 1 ppm of nitrogen dioxide (4 times the 1-hour California standard), 3 ppm of nitric oxide, and 4 ppm of carbon monoxide. The recommendations given for kerosene heaters apply to gas-fired space heaters.

Wood-Burning Stoves and Fireplaces

The few studies of wood-burning combustion sources that have been completed show that pollutants emitted include carbon monoxide, nitrogen oxides, hydrocarbons, and respirable particulates, including benzo-*a*-pyrene. Measurements show that pollutant emission rates from wood combustion vary over a wide range. The amount of carbon monoxide, nitrogen oxides, and particulates emitted by burning wood can vary by 100 times, depending on the amount of oxygen available and the burn temperature.

Although wood-burning stoves and fireplaces are vented to the outside, a number of circumstances can allow combustion products into the indoors: improper installation, cracks in the stovepipe, downdrafts, and spillage of wood from the fireplace. Little is currently known about the impact of wood burning on indoor air quality other than the obvious: that combustion products of wood are highly irritating to the eyes, nose, and respiratory system. However, several ongoing studies should increase our knowledge of this subject in the near future.

A wood-burning stove works differently from a fireplace. In a fireplace, as much as 90 percent of the fire's heat is lost up the chimney along with the exhaust gases. In a stove, the air supply is controlled, and thus the rate of burning is also controlled. The more efficient wood-burning stoves deliver 60 percent of the heat they produce to the indoors.

In a typical wood-burning stove (Fig. 5.5), room air enters through an

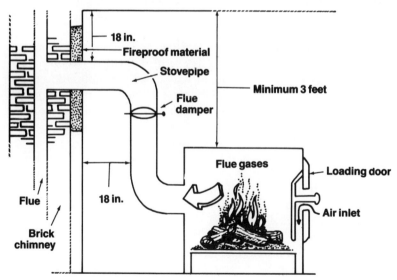

Fig. 5.5.   Installation and operation of a wood-burning stove.

opening whose size can be adjusted to regulate the rate at which the wood burns. The burning wood gives off both heat and combustion products. These combustion products pass through the flue pipe and into the chimney. A flue damper in the flue pipe can be used to fine-tune the fire or quench it if the stove overheats.

Wood-burning stoves are capable of producing from 10,000 to 50,000 BTU per hour. A gallon of fuel oil burned in a typical home furnace provides about 100,000 BTU to the house. In many homes, wood-burning stoves are used not as primary heat sources but for supplementary heat.

A field monitoring program designed to compare indoor and outdoor air pollution at ten residences was undertaken by Geomet Technologies, Inc., in the Boston metropolitan area.[23] Three of the residences used either a wood-burning stove or fireplace. Measurements indicated that wood burning produced elevated levels of total suspended particulates (TSP), respirable suspended particulates (RSP—defined in this study as particulates less than 3.5 micrometers in size), and benzo-*a*-pyrene. Average indoor TSP concentrations while the fire was lit were about three times their levels without the fire. The EPA standard was exceeded once during fireplace use.

Likewise, indoor concentrations of benzo-*a*-pyrene were five times higher when a wood-burning stove was in use. Although there is currently no health standard for benzo-*a*-pyrene, it is a known carcinogen, and any exposure above local background levels should be avoided if possible. Figure 5.6 shows indoor and outdoor concentrations in a residence with a wood-burning stove: during wood burning, indoor levels of benzo-*a*-pyrene ranged from 2 to 8 nanograms per cubic meter. Outdoor concentrations in heavily industrialized American cities average 1 nanogram per cubic meter on an annual basis; a comparable statistic for U.S. rural areas is about one-tenth that.[24] The residence with the wood-burning stove, otherwise an all-electric home, had an average infiltration rate of 0.68 ach, which is typical for existing homes. It is important to note that the stove was located in the basement immediately beneath the living room, where the air was sampled. Pollutant levels would have been higher if the room holding the stove had been sampled.

From this study and others, it is known that burning wood may lead to elevated indoor concentrations of particulates and nitrogen oxides that could be a significant factor in human exposure. This source of indoor air pollution may be particularly important in the less developed countries, as we saw in the case of India.

In this chapter, we have evaluated the indoor air quality impact of the following combustion appliances: gas stoves, kerosene- and gas-fired

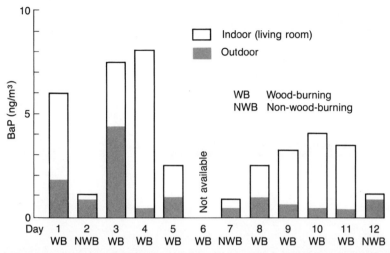

Fig. 5.6. Indoor and outdoor 24-hour concentrations of benzo-*a*-pyrene (BaP, in nanograms per cubic meter) in a residence with a wood-burning stove. Source: D. J. Moschandreas, J. Zabransky, and H. E. Rector, "The Effects of Woodburning on the Indoor Residential Air Quality," *Environment International*, vol. 4 (1980). Reprinted with permission from Pergamon Press, Ltd., and the author.

space heaters, and wood-burning stoves and fireplaces. It has been established that for homes using gas stoves and fans, a large percentage of combustion products can be exhausted to the outside before they are dispersed throughout the house. The exhaust fan should be used whenever the top burners or oven is operated. Unvented kerosene or gas-fired space heaters should be used only in well-ventilated areas or in large rooms for short periods of time. Wood-burning appliances are potential sources of particulates (in particular, benzo-*a*-pyrene) and nitrogen dioxide. Wood-burning stoves should be carefully installed, and all exhaust pathways should be periodically inspected for possible air leakage. A proper draft will help to exhaust combustion products efficiently. Since fireplaces are usually used for decorative or aesthetic purposes and burn wood only occasionally, the total exposure a house occupant will receive from their use should not be problematic unless they are used incorrectly with a poor draft.

6

Involuntary Smoking

Donna Shimp worked in an area of the New Jersey Bell Telephone Company where other employees smoked cigarettes. Finding herself to be allergic to cigarette smoke, Shimp sought an injunction requiring the employer to ban smoking on the job and eventually won her case in 1976 before the Superior Court of New Jersey.[1] This case set a precedent for common-law protection of nonsmokers' rights. Other plaintiffs have followed Shimp's footsteps in demanding smoke-free working environments. The city of San Francisco passed an ordinance in 1983 requiring private businesses to satisfy any employee's demand for a smoke-free work area. Despite some controversy when it was enacted, the ordinance took effect on schedule without incident.

A recent nationwide survey revealed that approximately 15 percent of U.S. businesses have programs to encourage and assist their employees to quit smoking. For example, Cybertek Computer Products, Inc., a Los Angeles software company, offers employees a $500 "health bonus" to quit smoking for a year. At Neon Electric Corporation in Houston, reformed smokers get a $.50 per hour raise after 6 months of not smoking.[2]

There are several reasons why these companies are discouraging smoking on the job. Employers realize that smokers directly cost them money through increased absenteeism, medical care, lost production time, and disability. Furthermore, several studies have now indicated that nonsmokers exposed to cigarette smoke suffer some of the same health hazards as light smokers. Finally, nonsmokers annoyed by cigarette smoke have one more reason to quit their jobs. William L. Weiss, of the Seattle University School of Business, conducted a year-long study into the cost of maintaining a smoker in the workplace. He concluded that a business loses $5,600 per year per smoker and that $560 of that loss is due to adverse health effects experienced by nonsmokers exposed to cigarette smoke on the job.[3]

Tobacco smoke is quite prevalent in indoor environments. Thirty percent of persons between the ages of 17 and 64 smoke cigarettes regularly. The results of three surveys in eight cities showed that the percentage of homes with one or more smokers ranged from 54 to 76 percent.[4] Since most of these homes had children, and since adults of child-bearing age are more likely to smoke, these percentages may be higher than for the average home. In addition, people are exposed to smoke at work and at other activities. The phenomenon of being exposed to other people's smoke is known as passive or involuntary smoking.

Components of Tobacco Smoke

The chemical constituents found in an atmosphere filled with tobacco smoke are derived from two sources, mainstream and sidestream smoke. Mainstream smoke is what the smoker inhales, then releases to the rest of the room. Sidestream smoke rises directly from the burning tobacco. Sidestream smoke is more important to the involuntary smoker because most of the time a cigarette is lit it produces only sidestream smoke, and because the combustion temperature is different. Over 2,000 chemical compounds have been identified in tobacco smoke; at least 40 of these are known to be carcinogens.

Some of the more important pollutants arising from tobacco smoke are carbon monoxide, benzo-*a*-pyrene, nicotine, nitrosamines, aldehydes, and acrolein. Acrolein and acetaldehyde both contribute to eye irritation. Nicotine, the active ingredient of tobacco leaves, may be the most important acute-acting toxic agent in tobacco smoke. Nicotine increases heart rate and blood pressure, and nicotine itself may be a significant carcinogen. The carcinogenic potency of cigarette tar appears to depend on its nicotine content. Benzo-*a*-pyrene, also a constituent of tar, is both carcinogenic and toxic.

Table 6.1 lists some of the compounds found in cigarette smoke and compares the total amount released from mainstream and sidestream smoke of one cigarette. As can be seen from the last column, showing the ratio of the amount of each compound found in sidestream smoke to the amount in mainstream smoke, sidestream smoke produces the greater quantity of each compound listed.

One substance not listed is polonium, a radioactive element that may contribute to lung and other cancers in smokers, owing to its emission of radiation within the body.[5] The amount of polonium found in tobacco

Table 6.1. Comparison of Mainstream and Sidestream Cigarette Smoke

Compound	Mainstream (mg/cig)	Sidestream (mg/cig)	Ratio side/main
Tar, no filter	20.8	44.1	2.1
Tar, filter	10.2	34.5	3.4
Nicotine, no filter	0.92	1.69	1.8
Nicotine, filter	0.46	1.27	2.8
Benzo-*a*-pyrene	0.000035	0.000135	3.7
Pyrene	0.00013	0.00039	3.0
Total phenols	0.228	0.603	2.6
Cadmium	0.000125	0.00045	3.6
Ammonia	0.16	7.4	46.0
Carbon monoxide	31.4	148.0	4.7
Nitrogen oxides	0.014	0.05	3.6
Hydrogen cyanide	0.24	0.16	3.6

SOURCE: *The Health Consequences of Smoking*, report of the Surgeon General (Washington, DC: U.S. Department of Health and Human Services, Public Health Services, 1981).

leaves varies with the place where the tobacco was grown. Polonium forms by the decay of radium, found in varying concentrations in soil, and by the decay of radioactive lead in the phosphate fertilizer used to grow tobacco.

Indoor Concentrations of Particulates from Smoke

Cigarette smoking in enclosed spaces increases the concentration of particulates, many of which are toxic. Measurements undertaken by James Repace, of the Environmental Protection Agency, and Alfred Lowrey, of the Naval Research Laboratory, showed that particulate concentrations in public buildings are often greater in magnitude than the 24-hour EPA air quality standard (260 micrograms per cubic meter) where smokers are present.[6] Table 6.2 lists the indoor and outdoor concentrations of respirable suspended particulates and the number of occupants smoking in some of these buildings. The presence of smokers caused RSP concentrations to be three to twelve times higher indoors than outdoors. Many of these particulates are small enough to penetrate down to the alveoli. The indoor concentrations were obtained over short time periods (usually less than 30 minutes), so they are not fully comparable to the 24-hour average that EPA standards regulate. The 24-hour average RSP concentration that a typical person would be exposed to is less than the values reported by Repace, assuming that some time would be spent in a smoke-free atmosphere. Nevertheless, the health standard is based on preventing adverse health effects from exposure to particulates found in outside air, and cigarette smoke particulates such as benzo-*a*-pyrene and nicotine may be more toxic than the typical particles found in outside air.

Table 6.2. Field Survey of Indoor Respirable Suspended Particulates (RSP)

Location	Number of occupants	Number of smokers	Indoor RSP ($\mu g/m^3$)	Outdoor RSP ($\mu g/m^3$)
Cocktail party	14	2	350	[a]
Lodge hall	350	40	700	60
Bar and grill	75	9	590	63
Pizzeria	50	5	415	40
Church				
Bingo game	150	20	280	[a]
Services	300	0	30	[a]
Bowling alley	128	14	200	50
Hospital waiting room	19	2	190	58

SOURCE: J. L. Repace and A. H. Lowrey, "Indoor Air Pollution, Tobacco Smoke, and Public Health," *Science*, vol. 208 (May 2, 1980). Copyright 1980 by the AAAS.

[a] Outdoor measurements were not taken.

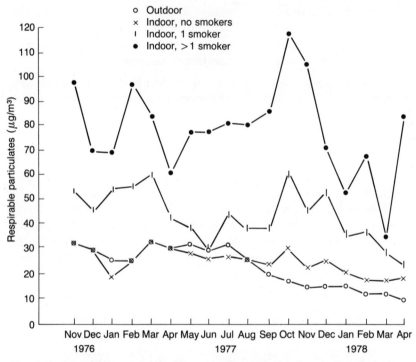

Fig. 6.1. Monthly mean respirable particulate concentration averaged over six U.S. cities. Source: J. D. Spengler *et al.*, "Long-Term Measurements of Respirable Sulfates and Particles Inside and Outside Homes," *Atmospheric Environment*, vol. 15 (1981). Reprinted by permission of the author.

Researchers from the Harvard School of Public Health monitored the concentration of respirable particulates in 80 residential buildings in six different U.S. cities.[7] Figure 6.1 shows the monthly average particulate concentrations over a 3-year period for all six cities. Daily indoor respirable particulate concentrations frequently exceeded 200 micrograms per cubic meter in homes with cigarette smokers. Respirable particulates were essentially the same indoors and outdoors in the homes without smokers, but indoor concentrations in homes with one or two cigarette smokers were two or three times higher. The annual average particulate concentration in homes with two or more smokers was 70 micrograms per cubic meter, close to the EPA 1-year standard of 75 micrograms per cubic meter.

These two studies indicate that involuntary smoking produces a significant particulate burden for people living in homes with smokers or spending much time in restaurants, bars, and other public buildings with smokers present. Few studies have looked at the constituents of this large category of pollutants, but significant amounts of benzo-*a*-pyrene and nicotine, both toxic materials, have been identified.

Indoor Concentrations of Carbon Monoxide from Smoke

Levels of carbon monoxide, a major product of tobacco combustion, have been studied in a variety of situations. Concentrations ranging from 2 to 110 ppm have been measured, depending on the size of the space in which the smoking occurs, the number and type of tobacco products smoked, and the amount of ventilation. Only under conditions of unusually heavy smoking and poor ventilation did carbon monoxide levels exceed the 8-hour EPA standard of 35 ppm. However, even in cases where the ventilation was considered adequate, carbon monoxide levels often exceeded the 1-hour EPA standard of 9 ppm. One must be careful when using these levels of carbon monoxide as measures of individual exposure because it is the carbon monoxide actually absorbed by the body that causes the harmful effects. This absorption varies from person to person, depending on factors such as duration of exposure, rate of breathing, and cardiorespiratory function.

Several investigators have measured changes in carboxyhemoglobin levels in nonsmokers exposed to smoke-filled environments. In some of these studies, the levels in nonsmokers rose slightly above 2 percent. A recent survey by the National Center for Health Statistics found that nonsmokers have an average carboxyhemoglobin level of about 1 percent and smokers have an average of greater than 4 percent.[8] A carboxyhemoglobin level above 2 percent in healthy nonsmokers is considered to be a potential health hazard. Increases of this magnitude are probably functionally insignificant in the healthy adult, but in persons with angina pectoris, any reduction of oxygen carrying capacity is of great importance. In this disease, the volume of blood able to be pumped through the coronary artery cannot meet the demands of the heart muscle under the stress of exercise. Research on persons with angina pectoris showed that the amount of exercise that could be performed before chest pain developed was significantly shortened after carbon monoxide exposure. This change occurred after a 2-hour exposure to 50 ppm of carbon monoxide and with an increase in carboxyhemoglobin level from 1 percent to 2.7 percent; this level is within the range produced by involuntary smoking.

Children's Health in Families with Smokers

Many studies have been undertaken to determine the effects of parental cigarette smoking on the health of their children; most found an adverse effect.[9] Two of these studies will be described; one found an increase in respiratory illness and the second a decrease in pulmonary function among such children.

The first was a study performed by the National Center for Health Statistics.[10] Data were collected on almost 67,000 children during interviews with parents by personnel of the U.S. Bureau of the Census. Data about illness and injury during the 2 weeks prior to the interview were collected for all ages. Children in families with no smokers had an average of fewer restricted-activity days (1 per year) and bed-disability days (0.8 per year) than did children in families with two smokers. Children in families with one smoker were in between the two other groups. Acute respiratory illness accounted for the difference in disability days. Family smoking was also measured by the combined number of cigarettes smoked by adults; children in families that smoked 45 or more cigarettes a day had 2 more restricted-activity days and 1 more bed-disability day per year due to acute respiratory illness than did children in families who did not smoke. The differences in disability days could not be explained by differences in education of the family head, children's age, family income, or the number of adults in the household.

One way in which the cigarette smoking of adults could make their children more susceptible to respiratory disease is by decreasing their lung functioning. The study described below looked at the relationship between lung function in children and parental cigarette smoking. Cigarette smoking by adults could affect their children's health by exposing the children to more disease if the smokers themselves have a higher incidence of disease. For example, the more often parents are ill with bronchitis, the more likely they are to transmit their infection to their children. This so-called clustering of respiratory illness has been searched for but not conclusively proved.

In the other study, researchers from Harvard Medical School examined the effect of parental smoking on the pulmonary function of their children aged 5 to 9 years.[11] A random sample of 444 Boston children was selected. Standardized questionnaires were used to obtain histories of respiratory symptoms and illness as well as smoking histories and demographic data. A spirometer recorded the amount of air the subjects could breathe out after taking a deep breath—the forced vital capacity, or FVC. The study found that the more smoking adults in a household, the greater the effect on the pulmonary function of their children. Comparing children in smoking and nonsmoking families yielded statistically insignificant results, but the pattern of decline in pulmonary function was consistent with *increased* family smoking in a statistically significant manner. The authors concluded, "Our findings suggest that a child's passive exposure to cigarette smoke has an adverse effect on the child's pulmonary function."

Involuntary Smoking in the Workplace

A large study of the effect of long-term voluntary smoking on certain indexes of pulmonary function in 2,100 middle-aged subjects also collected data on involuntary smoking at work.[12] Data were collected from people who had taken part in a physical fitness course sponsored by the Department of Physical Education at the University of California, San Diego. The subjects were divided into six groups ranging from nonsmokers not exposed to smoke to long-time heavy smokers. One of the groups consisted of nonsmokers exposed to smoke at work.

Table 6.3 summarizes the results of the forced expiratory flow (FEF) measurements for male and female smokers and nonsmokers. Many researchers believe that this quantity is more useful than forced vital capacity in early detection of small-airways obstruction. Airways in the respiratory system less than one-tenth inch in diameter are the sites where the obstructive process begins. Figure 6.2 illustrates the way in which FEF rates are calculated from a spirometer tracing. FEF (25–75%) is the rate of flow during the middle half of exhalation, between 25 and 75 percent of the total FVC. FEF (75–85%) is the rate of flow during the next 10 percent of the forced vital capacity. FEV-1 is the expiratory volume during the first second of exhalation.

Compared with the nonsmokers who worked in smoke-free environments, the subjects in the other five groups (see Table 6.3) had significantly lower values for FEF(25–75%) and FEF(75–85%). These lower

Table 6.3. Forced Expiratory Flow (FEF) Rates in Smokers and Nonsmokers

Group	Number of subjects	Sex	Percentage of predicted FEF (25–75%)	Percentage of predicted FEF (75–85%)
Nonsmokers, no smoke exposure	200	Female	108	112
	200	Male	104	120
Nonsmokers, smoke exposure at work >20 years	200	Female	93	85
	200	Male	91	95
Smokers, not inhaling	50	Female	92	85
	50	Male	92	87
Smokers inhaling 1–10 cig/day, >20 years	200	Female	89	83
	200	Male	89	77
Smokers inhaling 11–39 cig/day, >20 years	200	Female	78	69
	200	Male	76	68
Smokers inhaling ≥40 cig/day, >20 years	200	Female	72	62
	200	Male	72	60

SOURCE: J. R. White and H. F. Froeb, "Small-Airways Dysfunction in Nonsmokers Chronically Exposed to Tobacco Smoke," *New England Journal of Medicine*, vol. 302, no. 13 (March 1980). Reprinted by permission of the publisher.

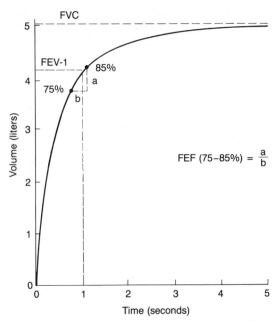

Fig. 6.2. A spirometer tracing illustrates forced vital capacity (FVC), forced expiratory volume in one second (FEV-1), and forced expiratory flow rate between 75 and 85 percent of the forced vital capacity (FEF(75–85%)).

levels are shown in Table 6.3 as percentages of predicted values according to the age and size of the subjects. The FVC and FEV-1 were not as sensitive. The involuntary smokers scored significantly lower than their nonsmoking counterparts; in fact, they were in the same state of impaired performance as the noninhalers and light smokers.

The authors of the study, James White and Herman Froeb, stated that the only substantial difference between the two nonsmoking groups is that the second was exposed to smoky workplace environments for a period of time greater than 20 years. The groups' occupations and working and living conditions were not significantly different. Eighty-three percent of the working subjects held professional, managerial, or technical positions, and the remainder were blue-collar workers. Most of the subjects lived in San Diego, an area low in air pollution. Candidates with health, environmental, or occupational conditions (besides smoking) that could influence pulmonary function adversely were disqualified from the study.

White and Froeb also stated that the traditional spirometric tests of forced vital capacity and forced expiratory volume are often normal in the presence of extensive small-airways disease. In contrast, the rates of mid-expiratory flow, FEF(25–75%), and end-expiratory flow, FEF(75–85%), reflect expiratory flow in the presence of smaller lung volumes during a period when airway segments may be in the process of closing. It can be concluded from this study that if long-term small-airways obstruction is occurring, nonsmokers who work in a smoky environment have about the same risk of impairment as do smokers who inhale between one and ten cigarettes a day. Further increases in exposure to cigarette smoke may cause a progression from small-airways obstruction to extensive bronchial and alveolar disease.

A recent French study came to the same conclusions as the White and Froeb study. A reduction in pulmonary function due to involuntary smoking at home was seen for adult women. Women with smoking husbands had significantly lower FVC, FEV-1, and FEF(25–75%).[13]

The short-term symptomatic effects of involuntary smoking are well documented.[14] The common complaints are eye, nose, and throat irritation, coughing, and sneezing. It is quite clear, from the health studies just described, that involuntary smoking also causes adverse health effects on the respiratory systems of children and adults. The possible association between involuntary smoking and lung cancer is much more controversial.

Involuntary Smoking and Lung Cancer

Lung cancer is a major health problem throughout most of the world. In the United States, more than 100,000 people die of lung cancer each

Table 6.4. Lung Cancer Death Rates Relative to Smoking Habits

Smoking habit	Number of men	Lung cancer deaths	Death rate (per 10^5 person-years)
Never smoked regularly	67,653	49	12
Current cigarette smokers			
1–9/day	23,072	26	56
10–19/day	39,690	82	90
20–39/day	115,930	381	159
40+/day	23,510	82	201

SOURCE: E. C. Hammond, *Smoking in Relation to the Death Rates of 100,000 Men and Women*, National Cancer Institute Monograph 19 (1966). By permission of the author.

year. Each year, some 100,000 Americans are told they have lung cancer; only about 10 percent will live another 5 years or more. The great majority of lung cancers are attributable to smoking.[15]

It has long been known that smoking increases the risk of contracting lung cancer and other diseases.[16] Among cigarette smokers, lung cancer death rates increase with the number of cigarettes smoked per day, degree of inhalation, and how young the smoker was when he or she began smoking. Results from a large American epidemiological study illustrate how lung cancer death rates increase with the number of cigarettes smoked per day.[17] At the start of the study, the men were aged 35 to 84 years. Deaths from lung cancer were recorded over a 4-year period. It can be seen from Table 6.4 that there is a steady increase in the death rate from lung cancer with increasing cigarette smoking. Compared to nonsmokers, men who smoke 20–39 cigarettes per day have thirteen times the mortality rate from lung cancer.

Does involuntary exposure to cigarette smoke increase the risk of contracting lung cancer? This is a very difficult question to answer because the dose of carcinogens received by involuntary smokers is small and hard to quantify in epidemiological studies. Three recent health studies attempted to answer this question.

The first study concluded that nonsmoking wives of heavy smokers have a higher risk of lung cancer than nonsmoking wives of nonsmoking husbands.[18] Takeshi Hirayama, chief of the Epidemiology Division of the National Cancer Research Institute in Tokyo, followed more than 90,000 nonsmoking housewives aged 40 and above for a period of 14 years and measured their risk of developing lung cancer according to the smoking habits of their husbands. It was assumed in this study that the wives received their main exposure to cigarette smoke from their husbands, since Japanese women tend not to work outside their homes.

Hirayama divided his study population into three groups: wives of nonsmokers, wives of ex-smokers or light to moderate smokers (1–19

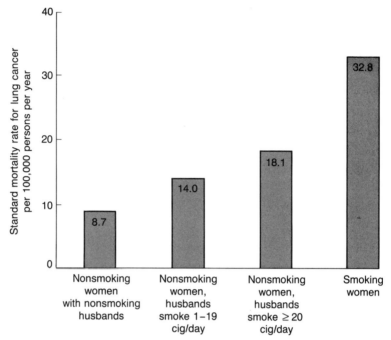

Fig. 6.3. Lung cancer mortality in women according to the presence or absence of direct and involuntary smoking. Source: T. Hirayama, "Nonsmoking Wives of Heavy Smokers Have a Higher Risk of Lung Cancer: A Study from Japan," *British Medical Journal*, vol. 282 (January 1981). By permission of the author and the *British Medical Journal*.

cigarettes per day), and wives of heavy smokers (20 or more cigarettes per day). Women whose husbands smoked more than 20 cigarettes per day were found to have twice the risk of lung cancer that wives of nonsmokers had. If the husbands smoked fewer than 20 cigarettes per day, the risk was 1.6 times higher than for the wives of nonsmokers.

The effect of involuntary cigarette smoking, as can be seen in Figure 6.3, was about one-half that of direct smoking. For example, the mortality rate for wives of light to moderate smokers was 14.0 per 100,000 persons per year, whereas the figure for women who smoked was 32.8 per 100,000. Smoking was the only habit of the husbands of all those studied (for example, alcohol consumption) that affected the wives' mortality rates. Hirayama concluded, "The fact that there was a statistically significant relationship between the amount the husbands smoked and the mortality of their nonsmoking wives from lung cancer suggests that these findings were not the result of chance." In countries such as Japan where many more men than women smoke (73 percent versus 15 percent), although the mortality risk from involuntary smoking is less than that from direct smoking, the number of deaths from lung cancer due to involuntary smoking may be important because of the large size of the exposed group (85 percent of all women are nonsmokers, and the majority are involuntarily exposed to tobacco smoke).

Several researchers commented on Hirayama's study after its publication in the *British Medical Journal*. One letter corroborated the Japanese study by referring to a Pennsylvania study that came to similar conclusions.[19] Another criticized the study because it did not take into account the exposure of Japanese women to indoor air pollution from household heating and cooking equipment,[20] which in Japan is often fueled by wood or kerosene. Smoke from wood fires has been suggested as a factor in lung cancer development, and cooking with kerosene stoves has been associated with lung cancer in women in Hong Kong.[21] If all Japanese women received the same exposure, this would not complicate the epidemiological study. However, there is some evidence that the more affluent have greater separation between living and cooking quarters and use electric heaters instead of wood or kerosene heaters. Another problem is that smoking habits may be related to social status, the more affluent smoking less. These two criticisms both fall under the category of not controlling for all important variables; in other words, the three population groups set up by Hirayama may not have been identical in every significant way.

Two other comments on Hirayama's work both concerned an alleged inconsistency in the subpopulation of unmarried women.[22] Certain assumptions were made by these critics in order to calculate a death rate for unmarried nonsmoking women, which is higher than that of nonsmoking wives of light to moderate smokers. They claim that 50 percent of unmarried women would have to smoke for this relationship to hold, whereas Hirayama's data showed that 34 percent of unmarried women smoke. It is also possible that unmarried women have greater exposure to·cigarette smoke outside the home than do married women. These comments underline how difficult it is to control all the variables that may influence health effects being considered in an epidemiological study. The need for several studies to reach similar conclusions is apparent.

The second study looking at the effect of involuntary smoking on the incidence of lung cancer was performed by D. Trichopoulos and his associates in Athens, Greece.[23] Fifty-one women with lung cancer and 163 other hospital patients (controls) were interviewed regarding their smoking habits and their husbands' or ex-husbands' smoking habits. Forty of the cancer patients and 149 of the controls were nonsmokers. Among these women, there was a higher risk of lung cancer when the husband smoked than when they had no exposure to cigarette smoke. If the husband smoked 1–19 cigarettes per day, their risk increased by 2.4 times; and if he smoked more than 20 cigarettes per day, the risk increased to 3.4 times that for women whose husbands did not smoke.

The third study examining the relationship between passive smoking and lung cancer was carried out by Pelayo Correa and associates in Louisiana.[24] It was found that nonsmokers married to heavy smokers (41 "pack-years" or more) had an increased risk of lung cancer. The number of cases was small, however: 10 males and 25 females of the 1,338 lung cancer patients were nonsmokers who had ever been married to heavy smokers. The increased risk of lung cancer for these passively exposed nonsmokers was twice as high as the rate for nonexposed people.

The accuracy of estimating a wife's exposure to cigarette smoke according to the smoking habits of her husband is questionable in general. However, it may be reasonable to assume that married women in Greece and Japan are segregated from men (other than husbands and brothers) to a far greater extent than in America. In conclusion, the three studies described indicate a similar effect: involuntary smoking significantly increases the incidence of lung cancer.

The American Tobacco Institute vigorously criticized Hirayama's study.[25] It pointed to the letters described above, omitting mention of the letter corroborating Hirayama's findings and ignoring Trichopoulos's study. However, a study by Lawrence Garfinkel, of the American Cancer Society, was cited as finding no significant increase in lung cancer among nonsmoking women married to smokers as compared to wives of nonsmokers.[26] Garfinkel's data showed a small increase in risk for wives of smokers but no increase with the number of cigarettes smoked by the husband, and the difference between wives of smokers and nonsmokers was not statistically significant. Garfinkel himself thinks that classifying nonsmoking women on the basis of their husbands' smoking habits is not an accurate method of determining exposure to cigarette smoke. Women's exposure to tobacco smoke outside the home may be very different in the United States from that in Japan and Greece. Until more research confirms or refutes the studies described above, it will be difficult to estimate the increased lung cancer risk experienced by involuntary smokers.

7

Energy-Efficient Buildings and Indoor Air Quality

More and more energy-efficient buildings have been built since the late 1970's. Rapidly escalating fuel prices that resulted in high heating and cooling bills increased consumer demand for such buildings. Initially, home builders and energy researchers focused on improving the energy efficiency of new buildings, but great energy savings possible from retrofitting old homes were neglected. The U.S. Department of Energy addressed this earlier imbalance by requiring electric and gas utilities to offer energy conservation assistance to their residential customers.

Despite concern by the Environmental Protection Agency because of potential adverse health effects, large-scale weatherization programs are being carried out by utilities across the country. Many consumers are installing insulation and tightening their homes against cold winter drafts. How effective are these measures in reducing energy use, and what adverse health effects was the EPA concerned about? This chapter will look at the various energy conservation measures and see how they decrease energy use. The effects of these measures on indoor air quality will be assessed.

Principles of Energy Efficiency

The basic purpose of constructing energy-efficient buildings is to keep warm air inside in the winter and cool air inside in the summer. The less energy needed for heating and cooling, the lower fuel bills will be. Most heat loss occurs through two mechanisms, conduction and infiltration (see Fig. 7.1). Some materials conduct heat better than others; because of the very poor heat conductivity of air, double-pane windows containing an air space will keep a house warmer in winter than two panes placed back to back. Heat loss from conduction depends on the heat conductivity of a house's materials and on the temperature difference across the roof, walls, and windows. The greater the temperature difference, the greater the heat loss. Infiltration is the air leakage through cracks and openings in the building; warm air leaving is replaced by an equal amount of incoming cold air that must be warmed up to the desired indoor temperature. Heat loss through leakage takes place by convection, or the transfer of heat by the motion of the heat-carrying fluid (a gas or liquid). Another example of convection is the movement of hot air up a chimney.

Measures to improve the energy efficiency of a residence involve decreasing heat losses by conduction and exfiltration. (Other methods include installing energy-efficient appliances and using solar energy for space or water heating.) Cutting heat flows can work in two ways, by saving heat energy in winter and by saving cooling expenses in summer.

Energy-efficient houses incorporate large quantities of insulation in their roof, walls, and floors. Heat loss through windows, which is also a significant fraction of total heat loss, can be reduced by using double- or triple-pane windows and drapes or insulating shutters. To reduce heat loss via exfiltration one can construct homes with tighter-fitting doors and windows, plug leaks in the building envelope with caulking compound, and install vapor barriers. A vapor barrier is usually a thin plastic sheet stretched across the exterior wall framing on all sides of a house beneath the ceiling joists, and under the subflooring. The vapor barrier

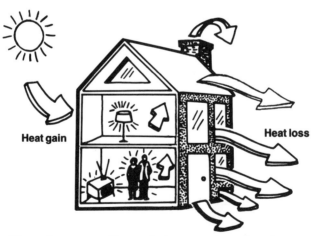

Fig. 7.1. The main sources of heat gain (sun, people, and appliances) and heat loss (conduction through roof, walls, and windows, and exfiltration) for a residential building during the winter.

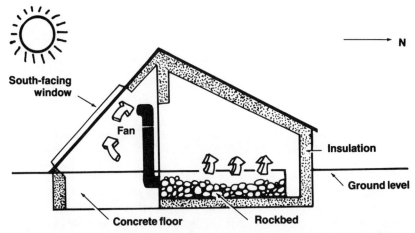

Fig. 7.2. During the day, solar radiation passes through a large south-facing window and heats up the south-facing room. Warm air is passed by a fan and ductwork through a rockbed, where heat energy is stored to be tapped during the cold night.

impedes the flow of water vapor and air through the building envelope, the net effect being to keep indoor air indoors for a longer time. Therefore, all else being equal, indoor-generated contaminants will reach higher concentrations in energy-efficient houses.

Another strategy for reducing home energy use may also affect the indoor air. Passive solar homes employ south-facing windows (see Fig. 7.2) to gather solar energy during the day and various means to store this energy for use at night. One type of storage system is composed of a bed of rocks; fans circulate sun-warmed air to the rockbed beneath the house. At night, air from the living spaces is warmed in the rockbed and circulated throughout the house. This type of storage system could present indoor air quality problems if the rocks emanate radon. No measurements have been made to evaluate this possibility, so little more can be said, but isolating the indoor air by piping it through the rockbed ought to prevent any problems.

Measurements of Air Quality in Energy-Efficient Residences

There is an obvious conflict between the goals of saving energy through reduced infiltration and maintaining indoor air quality. About one-third of the heat loss in the typical single-family home is through exfiltration of warm inside air to the cold outside. Reduction of infiltration (and thus exfiltration) usually causes the concentrations of indoor-generated con-

Table 7.1. Cost of Heating Infiltrating Air During the Winter

	Chicago		Washington, DC	
Utility	Energy use (therms)	Annual cost of fuel	Energy use (therms)	Annual cost of fuel
Natural gas	400	$160	280	$165
Oil	400	325	280	260
Electricity	260	600	180	345

SOURCE: W. J. Fisk and I. Turiel, "Residential Air to Air Heat Exchangers: Performance, Energy Savings and Economics," *Energy and Buildings*, vol. 5 (1983).

taminants to rise; this is one side of the conflict. On the other hand, reducing infiltration saves energy and money. Table 7.1 shows the cost of heating the air that infiltrates into typical 1,500-square-foot houses during the winter, assuming that the infiltration rate averages 0.75 air changes per hour. Whether the home is heated with gas, oil, or electricity, the cost of the energy lost to exfiltration amounts to hundreds of dollars a year. Are the savings offset by the threat of greater pollution indoors?

The Energy-Efficient Buildings Group at Lawrence Berkeley Laboratory has investigated indoor air quality in 36 energy-efficient residences.[1] About half were newly built; the rest were weatherized to be more energy efficient. A significant finding of this research is that indoor air quality depends more on the sources of air pollution present in or near the building than on the infiltration rate. The indoor air quality in low-infiltration buildings may be similar to that in typical buildings.

Many pollutants were measured during these studies, but only formaldehyde, nitrogen dioxide, and radon were extensively monitored. In 2 of the 36 homes, formaldehyde concentrations exceeded the 100 parts per billion (ppb) level of concern; new furniture appeared to be the source. All 36 homes were monitored for nitrogen dioxide, and one had an average nitrogen dioxide concentration greater than 50 ppb, the U.S. ambient air quality standard for annual average concentration; this house used a wood-burning stove for its space heating. Respirable suspended particulates (RSP) were measured in 18 homes; in 2 the RSP concentration was greater than 50 micrograms per cubic meter. This concentration is still below the long-term standards for particulates. Smokers were identified as the main source of RSP in both houses.

Radon was measured in 31 of the houses, and 2 had radon concentrations greater than the level of concern (3 to 4 nanocuries per cubic meter). In one, the radon level was extremely high—25 nanocuries per cubic meter. This measurement was in a house specially built by the National Association of Home Builders (NAHB) in Mt. Airy, Maryland, to demonstrate techniques for constructing energy-efficient homes. Although this home was extremely tight (0.15 air changes per hour average infiltration rate), that alone could not account for such a high concentration of radon.

After this discovery, additional measurements were made in the NAHB house and in 37 houses located within a mile or two of the NAHB house.[2] Once again, high radon concentrations were found in the NAHB home. Even though the infiltration rates were similar in the two samples (the 37 additional homes and the original 31 homes across the United States), the radon concentrations measured in the second sample were substantially different. Thirty percent of the measurements in the second sample, compared to 6.5 percent in the first sample, exceeded 4 nanocuries per cubic meter. The difference in these two samples is probably due to the fact that radon source strengths were greater in the Mt. Airy area than for the nationwide sample. It is probable that the local geological properties of the soil surrounding a house are the major factor in determining indoor radon concentrations; also important are effective transport processes by which radon from nearby soil is brought indoors.

In summary, this limited study indicates that low-infiltration, energy-efficient homes do not, in general, have indoor air quality problems. Sources of pollutants and the presence of effective transport processes are the main determinants of indoor air pollutant levels in homes. There is generally no major difference between pollutant sources in energy-efficient and conventional homes, except for homes that may have been weatherized with urea-formaldehyde foam insulation, in which case formaldehyde levels tend to be higher than in conventional homes. In most cases, concentrations of indoor-generated pollutants can be expected to be somewhat higher in energy-efficient homes, but if significant sources of pollutants are not present, concentrations will not usually reach hazardous levels in either house type. It should be noted that this is a limited sample of energy-efficient homes and that organics (other than aldehydes) and water vapor were not sampled.

Low-infiltration homes tend to be subject to higher humidity, owing to the retention of indoor-generated water vapor. There are several potential adverse effects on building materials resulting from the increased humidity. Water vapor can condense on cold surfaces such as the walls of unheated attics or on window frames, which could lead to dry rot, faster deterioration of wood members, or paint damage if dripping occurs. Mildew and mold may also result from increased humidity indoors, owing to increased growth of fungi on fabrics and walls. Aside from the damage to exposed surfaces, there is an unpleasant odor associated with mildew.

Utility Weatherization Programs

The National Energy Conservation Policy Act of 1978 directed the U.S. Department of Energy to establish a conservation program for utilities.[3] The objective was to encourage people to adopt energy-conservation measures and to utilize renewable resources by retrofitting existing residential buildings. Under the act, gas and electric utilities were required to offer on-site energy audits to identify potential savings and estimated costs of conservation measures. The consumer can decide whether to carry out the conservation measures described in the audit.

Gas and electric utility companies are now offering free or low-cost energy audits and financial incentives to encourage their customers to weatherize. In many states, low-interest loans are available to consumers who wish to weatherize their homes. There is also a federal income tax credit for certain energy-conservation measures. Some utility companies, such as northern California's Pacific Gas and Electric, offer zero-interest loans to consumers. The California program, called ZIP (zero-interest program) for short, offers a $1,000 no-interest loan for six energy-conservation measures: insulating water heaters, installing low-flow shower heads, installing attic insulation, weatherstripping, caulking leaks, and insulating heating ducts in unheated rooms. More money ($2,500) is available for other conservation measures if an energy audit shows they are cost-effective. These measures include installing wall and floor insulation, storm doors and windows, and electronic ignition devices for gas appliances.

A 10-year weatherization program of the Bonneville Power Administration (BPA) is expected to cost $500 million.[4] The BPA is a federal agency that acquires power resources and then sells electricity to local utilities in Washington, Oregon, Idaho, and western Montana. They are required to promote energy conservation and renewable resources where the cost is less than that of electricity from new nuclear or coal-fired power plants. The financial incentive in the BPA program is a cash payment, based on the estimated energy savings, when the weatherization measures are completed and inspected. Certain measures that reduce infiltration are not offered to all customers, only to those in homes where the BPA feels indoor air quality degradation is not a serious issue. Homes with unvented space heaters, wood-burning stoves, and urea-formaldehyde foam insulation are on the exclusion list, unless the homeowner buys an air-to-air heat exchanger. Most utilities have not established criteria for excluding certain homes from their weatherization programs.

A number of homes have been weatherized by scientists in the Energy Efficient Buildings Program at Lawrence Berkeley Laboratory.[5] Analysis of data from three cities (Midway, Washington; Medford, Oregon; and Walnut Creek, California) shows that an infiltration rate reduction of 25 to 30 percent is typical, although the reduction may vary from 0 to 60 percent. For many nonreactive pollutants, a 25 to 30 percent reduction in infiltration rate results in an equivalent increase in the concentration of indoor-generated pollutants. An important exception is formaldehyde: a 25 percent reduction in infiltration rate results in a lesser increase in formaldehyde concentration. If no significant sources of indoor air pollution are present, this increase in concentration of indoor air pollutants will generally not cause any adverse health effects. However, residences with high levels of radon, formaldehyde, or combustion products should not have their infiltration rates reduced.

Tightening Residences

Air leakage increases the heating load on a furnace and on the heating bill as well, as Table 7.1 showed. A well-sealed house, in addition to saving money, is more comfortable because there are fewer cold drafts in winter. In addition, tightening a house often helps to maintain a more comfortable humidity level in the winter by keeping more moisture inside.

Figure 7.3 illustrates air leakage sites in a typical house. Air enters

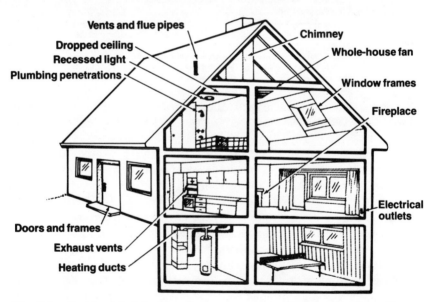

Fig. 7.3. Residential air leakage sites are numerous. Source: *The House Doctor's Manual*, Lawrence Berkeley Laboratory Publication 3017, prepared for the Department of Energy (Washington, DC: Government Printing Office, 1981).

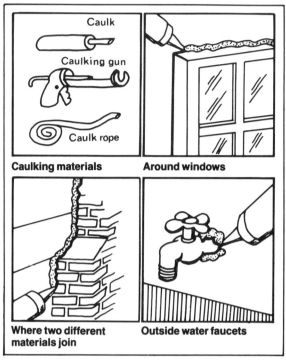

Use a solvent or a small chisel to free area to be caulked of dirt, loose paint, and deteriorated caulk. Cut the nozzle of the cartridge at a 45° angle. Some cartridges have an inner seal that will need to be punctured with a long nail. When caulking, hold the gun parallel to the joint at a 45° angle. Large cracks should first be stuffed with oakum or similar packing material.

Fig. 7.4. How and where to caulk. Source: *Find and Fix the Leaks*, Lawrence Berkeley Laboratory Publication 384, prepared for the Department of Energy (Washington, DC: Government Printing Office, 1981).

through cracks and leaky joints in the exterior walls of the building and around doors, windows, chimneys, or any other opening. Any penetration in the building envelope, such as for plumbing or electricity, is a likely source of air infiltration. Wherever different materials come together they can shrink and pull apart, causing leaks, as around the foundation seal. Caulking (Fig. 7.4) and weatherstripping (Fig. 7.5) will seal most leaks if done carefully, as explained in any home-care book.[6]

Weatherstripping doors and windows and caulking leaky places in the building envelope are productive steps in tightening a house, but they will not stop every leak. That goal may be closely approached as part of a procedure known as "house doctoring," a combination of energy audit and energy-saving retrofit procedures developed at Lawrence Berkeley Laboratory and Princeton University.

House doctoring analyzes areas of energy loss in which economically attractive conservation investments can be made, but goes beyond a conventional audit by locating and eliminating air infiltration sites. Several diagnostic tools are used to locate the leaks in a house, most notably infrared scanners and smokesticks. An infrared scanner is a hand-held device that is essentially an infrared video camera. When pointed at an object it shows warm spots as bright areas. It can be used to check the attic floor for "hot spots," places where the insulation blanket is inadequate and warm air is flowing up from below. Smokesticks can be used to trace air currents flowing through openings in the floor and around pipes, vents, and light fixtures.

House doctoring is more time-consuming than a typical weatherization procedure. It takes two people about 3 hours to install attic insulation, weatherstrip doors and windows, and perform minimal caulking, whereas house doctoring may take those two people a full day for infiltration-reducing measures alone. It is questionable whether house doctoring is a cost-effective procedure for decreasing energy use in resi-

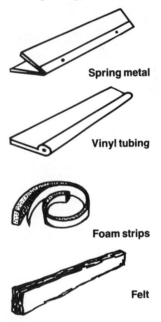

Spring metal or plastic weatherstripping consists of strips of metal or plastic in a V-shape. It is used for compression seals and sliding seals, typically where the bottom of the window sash contacts the window frame or in the channels of a window frame. Spring weatherstripping must be nailed or bonded to the window or door frame. Although moderately expensive, it is generally very durable.

Spring metal

Vinyl tubing comes in both reinforced and unreinforced form. Reinforced tubing contains a metal strip that keeps the tubing stiff. This type of weatherstripping can be used for compression and sliding seals. It is generally nailed to the window frame or doorframe. It does not cost very much and lasts 2 to 3 years. Vinyl tubing is also available with a magnetic core for use on metal doors.

Vinyl tubing

Foam strips come in open- or closed-cell form, and are backed by adhesive. (The adhesive on foam strips is generally inadequate, making it wise to tack or nail the strips in place.) Foam is best used for compression seals. It is inexpensive and usually lasts a few years.

Foam strips

Felt, which comes in reinforced and unreinforced form, does not cost very much. It is often used for compression seals, but has an effective lifetime of only 1 to 2 years. It must be tacked in place.

Felt

Fig. 7.5. The four types of weatherstripping. Source: *The House Doctor's Manual,* Lawrence Berkeley Laboratory Publication 3017, prepared for the Department of Energy (Washington, DC: Government Printing Office, 1981).

dential buildings. The usual weatherization measures listed earlier in this chapter are cost-effective in most parts of the United States.

Is it safe to tighten houses as recommended by local utilities? Typically, windows and doors will be weatherstripped and large obvious cracks or openings in the building envelope will be caulked. As discussed earlier, the average house will have a 25 to 30 percent reduction in infiltration rate. Unless significant sources of indoor air pollution are present, it should be safe to go ahead with these house-tightening measures.

Homeowners with high radium concentrations in the soil (and thus potentially high indoor radon levels) should not participate in house tightening. But other energy-conservation measures may be undertaken. The local utility may know of radon measurements taken in the area; if not, there are firms that can make such measurements (see Appendix B). Homes with urea-formaldehyde foam in the walls or with large amounts of relatively new particle board or plywood should probably not be tightened either. Again, private companies can make measurements of formaldehyde concentration if the local utility will not do so (see Appendix B). Homes with unvented space heaters should not be tightened. Homes with gas stoves may be tightened if a range hood is used over the stove.

Certain other situations lie in a gray area, and the individual homeowner must decide what course of action to take. Examples are homes where the occupants smoke or where wood-burning stoves or fireplaces are used frequently. These are intermittent sources of indoor air pollutants, and one can increase ventilation when these devices are used to compensate for the reduction in infiltration caused by house tightening. (Actually, infiltration automatically increases, owing to natural convection currents set up when a fireplace or wood-burning stove is in operation and using indoor air for combustion.)

Some utilities (for example, those in the BPA region) will take a limited inventory of potential sources of indoor air pollutants if requested before weatherization; currently, most utilities do not. Until they do, it is up to consumers to educate themselves on the issues discussed in this chapter.

8

Control of Indoor Air Pollutants

Previous chapters discussed several methods of reducing the concentration of specific indoor air contaminants: formaldehyde and radon were two. Here we take a general approach to the control of indoor air pollutants. There are three general methods of contaminant control: source removal or alteration, ventilation, and air cleaning.

Source Alteration or Substitution

Source removal is the ideal method of controlling indoor air contaminants. It is a permanent measure that requires no future operating or maintenance costs for it to remain effective. This method applies to situations where the source is known (for example, cigarette smoke) and a substitute is not required (see Fig. 8.1). Substitution is a more common method of source control. The source of a contaminant is removed from a dwelling and replaced by a cleaner device with the same basic function. An example is the use of an electric stove in place of a gas stove. A source may also be altered by a change in design to have a lower emission, for example, using an electric ignition rather than a gas pilot light in gas stoves. The figure shows several other source control methods. These include encapsulation—sealing off the source—and spatial confinement—walling it off. Finally, timing the production of contaminants to periods when occupancy of a dwelling is at a minimum also reduces exposure.

Ventilation

The concentration of contaminants may be reduced by local ventilation (for example, with an exhaust fan, discussed in Chapter 5) or by

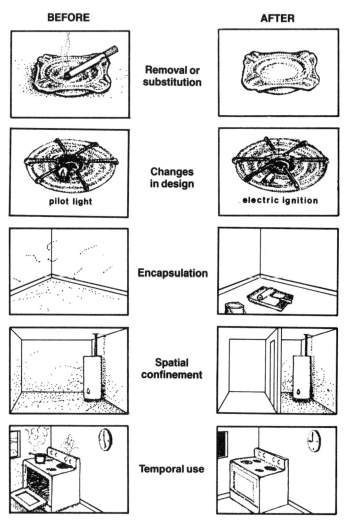

BEFORE ... **AFTER**

Removal or substitution

Changes in design — pilot light / electric ignition

Encapsulation

Spatial confinement

Temporal use

Fig. 8.1. The main methods of contaminant source control. Source: *Indoor Air Quality Handbook* (Albuquerque, NM: Sandia National Laboratories and Ana-Chem, Inc., 1982).

general air exchange between inside and outside air (see Fig. 8.2). Air exchange reduces pollutant levels by replacing indoor air with outside air, which works well when the outside air is cleaner. It is effective for all contaminant types. The drawback is that, depending on the climate, large quantities of incoming air may have to be heated or cooled. In good weather, opening windows is an effective, free method of contaminant control that should not be ignored merely because it is simple.

If the energy costs of ventilation are significant, a remedy may lie in ventilation with heat recovery. A heat exchanger can retain most of the heat normally lost when warm inside air (in the winter) is exhausted to the outside. Heat exchangers are commonly used in tightly built Swedish houses. They are cost-effective when used in cold parts of the United States.[1]

A residential heat exchanger generally consists of a core, two fans, and two filters all mounted in an insulated case (see Fig. 8.3). One fan brings outdoor air (supply air) through the core and into the house; the second fan pulls an equal amount of house air (exhaust air) through the core and out of the house. As the air passes through the core, heat is transferred across a thin partition from the warmer to the cooler airstream (usually without the two airstreams making contact). Thus (in the winter), the supply air is warmed before entering the house, and the exhaust air is cooled before leaving the house. The reverse process can keep the heat outside in the summer.

Most models of residential heat exchangers use a duct system for air distribution and can often be connected to existing ductwork where a

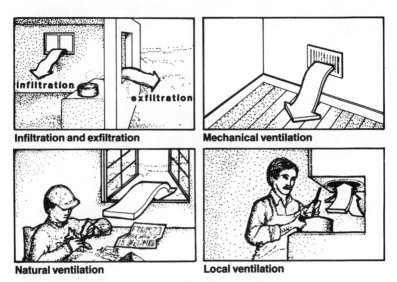

Fig. 8.2. Various types of ventilation can be used to remove contaminants from the air. Source: *Indoor Air Quality Handbook* (Albuquerque, NM: Sandia National Laboratories and AnaChem, Inc., 1982).

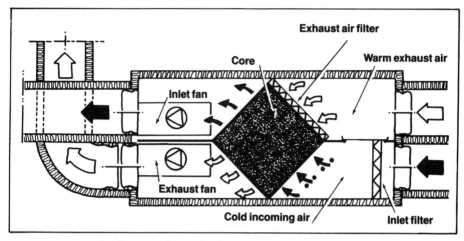

Fig. 8.3. A schematic diagram of an air-to-air heat exchanger. Source: W. J. Fisk *et al.*, *Freezing in Residential Air-to-Air Heat Exchanger: An Experimental Study,* Lawrence Berkeley Laboratory Report LBL-16783 (1983).

central heating system is employed. In homes with electrical-resistance strip heating, window or wall units, roughly the size of a window air conditioner, may be installed. The cost of a residential heat exchanger ranges from $250 for a window unit to $750 for a larger unit. Several manufacturers are listed in Appendix B.

Air Cleaning

If indoor air pollution cannot be prevented, sealed off, or blown away, it can still be taken out of the air. There are several methods of cleaning air, that is, removing contaminants that have already been introduced into the air from their sources. These are filtration, absorption, adsorption, and electrostatic precipitation.

Filtration

Filters may be used to remove particles from an airstream (see Fig. 8.4). They are composed of porous materials such as fabric, paper, or charcoal. The factors important for characterizing the trapping ability of filters are the average fiber diameter, fiber packing density (or pore size), and airflow rate. Slow airflow and densely packed fibers give the highest particle collection efficiency.

The trapping ability of filters also varies with particle size. Large particles like pollen are easy to remove; the medium-sized respirable particles

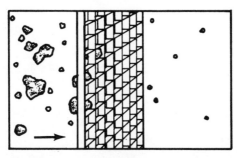

Fig. 8.4. Mechanical filters trap airborne particles. Source: *Indoor Air Quality Handbook* (Albuquerque, NM: Sandia National Laboratories and AnaChem, Inc., 1982).

of cigarette smoke are more difficult to trap; and even smaller particles are the hardest to trap. High-efficiency particulate air filters can remove almost all particles larger than 0.3 micrometer, which includes bacteria and spores but not viruses. Such filters are often used in hospital operating rooms, where the control of airborne microorganisms is critical. High-efficiency air filters have higher resistance to airflow and require more fan power to move air through them than the filters found in most air cleaners or in residential furnace systems. Fibrous mat filters, commonly used in furnaces, do not remove particulates of respirable size. Filters must be periodically cleaned or replaced, and trade-offs exist between filter cost, collection efficiency, and airflow resistance.

Absorption

Absorption processes have not been used for control of indoor air pollutants. Absorption is used industrially to control gaseous pollutants such as sulfur dioxide and nitrogen dioxide by passing a polluted airstream through a liquid in a thin layer on a solid surface. The pollutants dissolve in the liquid or react chemically with it; some particulates come out too. Water, with or without additives, is commonly used as the absorbent liquid.

Adsorption

Adsorbents are porous materials with a large surface area due to the presence of microscopic pores (Fig. 8.5). As gases pass through an adsorbent, they react through electrical forces with the molecules composing the adsorbent and cling to its surface. Adsorbents must be replaced periodically. Three commonly used adsorbents are activated charcoal, acti-

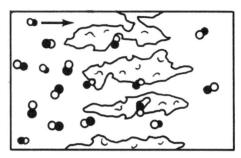

Fig. 8.5. Adsorption takes place when gas molecules attach themselves to the surface of an adsorbent material such as activated charcoal. Source: *Indoor Air Quality Handbook* (Albuquerque, NM: Sandia National Laboratories and Ana-Chem, Inc., 1982).

vated alumina, and silica gel. Large molecules are more easily trapped than small molecules, limiting the effectiveness of the method to organic gases of high molecular weight. There is some evidence that the adsorbent alumina oxide impregnated with potassium permanganate is effective in removing formaldehyde from indoor air.[2]

Electrostatic Precipitation

The physical principle behind electrostatic precipitation, or electronic air cleaning, is that positively and negatively charged particles attract each other. Airborne particles carried into the cleaner by a fan receive a positive charge as they pass through an electric field (see Fig. 8.6), then enter a second electric field between a series of metal plates. The positively charged particles are attracted to the negative plates, where they collect. The collection surfaces must be cleaned periodically, usually with soap and water. When properly maintained, electrostatic precipitators are effective in removing dust, smoke particles, and some allergens from room air.

Another electrostatic device is the air ionizer (see Fig. 8.7). These devices boost the 120-volt house current to as high as 20,000 volts and send it onto pointed metal needles, where the electric field imparts energy to nearby free electrons, in effect spraying ions into the air. When these ions collide with airborne particles they can impart some electrical charge to the particulates. Ionizers generally do not have a collection surface as do electrostatic precipitators; therefore, the charged particulates attach to the nearest indoor surface. The wall near an ionizer gradually develops a gray circle of grime—a consequence of air ionizer use not often made clear to users. Several manufacturers now offer units with collection sur-

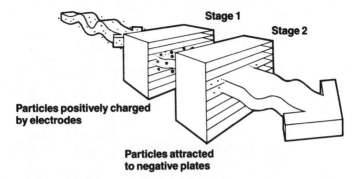

Fig. 8.6. A two-stage electrostatic precipitator. The first stage charges particles, and the second stage removes the particles from the airstream. Source: *Indoor Air Quality Handbook* (Albuquerque, NM: Sandia National Laboratories and AnaChem, Inc., 1982).

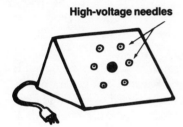

Fig. 8.7. A negative-ion generator produces negatively charged air ions. The unit is the size of a teapot.

faces. Since ionizers do not usually contain fans, they rely on general air circulation to bring particles to the ionization source.

Air Cleaners as Particulate Control Devices

The market for portable residential air cleaners is several years old, and already well over 10 million have been sold in this country. Some of these desktop air cleaners sell for as little as ten dollars. How well do these air-cleaning devices operate, and how well do they clean the indoor air? Since there is currently no standard testing procedure, there is little information on the performance of these air cleaners beyond the manufacturers' claims. The results of three independent studies indicate a wide range in performance.

Filters, electronic air cleaners, and ion generators can all be used to control airborne particulates; adsorbents are used for the control of gaseous pollutants. The air pollutant control devices described here were designed to stand alone, unconnected to central heating and cooling systems; connected devices are also available.

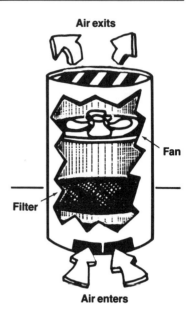

Air exits

Fan

Filter

Air enters

Fig. 8.8. In a fan-filter air-cleaning device, room air passes through a filter, where some of the particulates are trapped. Some units have adsorbents impregnated in the filter to control odors.

There are basically three types of residential air cleaners being sold: fan-filter units, electrostatic air cleaners, and negative-ion generators. A fan-filter device, the kind not yet discussed, is composed of a fan and filter housed inside a plastic case (see Fig. 8.8). Most units easily fit on a desk top. The fan draws room air through a replaceable filter, where some fraction of the airborne particulates is trapped. Many filters include chemically active ingredients such as charcoal or scented crystals to reduce odors. There are two possible processes going on at the same time here: charcoal or silica gel filters adsorb gaseous contaminants that are responsible for odors, and the scented ingredient masks other odors, such as cigarette smoke, with pleasing smells resembling citrus fruits.

The product-testing department of *New Shelter* magazine has tested twelve fan-filter air cleaners, five negative-ion generators, and one hybrid machine for their ability to remove particulates from the air.[3] They generated cigarette smoke in a room 13 by 12 by 8 feet and measured the concentration of particulates for a 4-hour period while operating the various air-cleaning devices. At the start of each test, the particulate concentration was 50 micrograms per cubic meter. A smoking machine was used to raise the particulate concentration to 1,000 micrograms per cubic meter; then each device was turned on in turn, and the effect on the concentration of particulates was recorded. All of the adjustable air cleaners were run at their highest setting. The test room was thoroughly cleaned between test runs.

The particles in cigarette smoke are quite small, typically less than 1 micrometer across. Pollen grains vary from about 10 to 100 micrometers, and for comparison's sake, human hairs are 30 to 200 micrometers thick. The smallest particulates pose the greatest health risk. These are the particles that reach the lungs and remain there for long times. Therefore, the choice of cigarette smoke particulates for these tests is reasonable, although it provides no information on the ability of the air cleaners to control larger or smaller particulates. Sound levels and ozone concentration were also measured (some negative-ion generators are thought to produce small quantities of ozone, which is a lung irritant).

Three tests were run without any air-cleaning device in the test room. On the average, after 4 hours, 17 percent of the smoke particulates settled out of the air or became attached to various surfaces, owing to gravity and natural air currents in the room. To denote the other extreme, a large, high-capacity air cleaner was tested. It was much more expensive ($300) than the other units and contained a fan, a prefilter, and a high-efficiency particulate air filter. It cleaned all the smoke from the room in 2 hours and 41 minutes.

Figure 8.9 shows the results for all the air cleaners tested. Their effectiveness in removing tobacco smoke is expressed as an effective clean-air flow rate, the flow rate of clean air that would produce the observed particulate decay rate. It is assumed that the reduction in the number of particulates occurs exponentially and that there is perfect mixing of the air in the test room. An effective clean-air flow rate of 5 cubic feet per minute (cfm) means that the rate of decrease for particulates is equivalent to that obtained if 5 cfm of clean outside air were to infiltrate into the test room. The negative-ion generators removed the smoke much faster than the fan-filter devices: four out of five removed 96 percent of the smoke in 4 hours or less, and the fifth removed 70 percent in 4 hours, better than the best fan-filter machine. The Orbit and Air Care II both have built-in particle collectors, unlike the other three. It should be noted that the effectiveness of the ion generators may have been exaggerated in these tests because small fans were used to keep the air well mixed. The fan-filter devices had almost the same effective clean-air flow rates, at least for cigarette smoke, as were obtained by doing nothing at all (leftmost bar). The ion generators are more costly (average $120) than the fan-filter units (average $35). Several manufacturers of air ionizers are listed in Appendix B.

A hybrid machine (the Biotech Bionaire 1000), a combination fan-filter device and ion generator, was the most effective smoke remover, removing all of the smoke in just 1 hour and 46 minutes. It has the highest clean-air flow rate (60 cfm). Its $250 price is higher than that of the other devices, but it had a 50 percent higher effective clean-air flow rate than

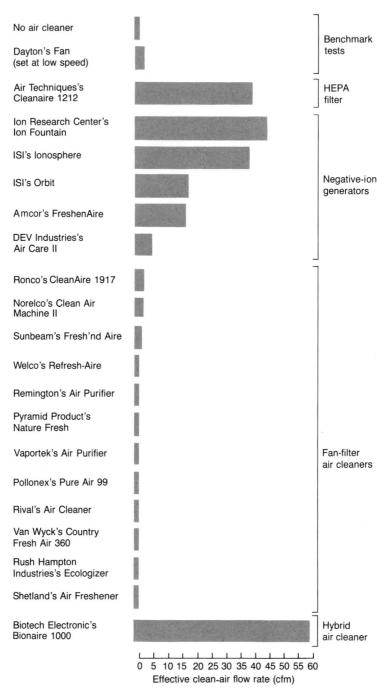

Fig. 8.9. A comparison of the performance of portable residential air cleaners in removing tobacco smoke, as reported in *New Shelter*, July–August 1982. HEPA, high-efficiency particulate air. Source: Lawrence Berkeley Laboratory.

the $300 high-efficiency filter. Interestingly, a simple floor fan removed 54 percent of the smoke in 4 hours, presumably by circulating particulates near surfaces where they attached themselves. The problem with this technique is that the particulates may become airborne again unless they are cleaned off of the walls, ceiling, floor, and furniture with a wet cloth.

None of the ion generators, including the hybrid machine, released any detectable amount of ozone. The sound tests showed that the fan-filter devices produced noise equivalent to that produced by light automobile traffic at a distance of 100 feet. The air ionizers were silent.

Researchers at Lawrence Berkeley Laboratory tested ten portable residential air cleaners in a room 11 by 13.5 by 8 feet.[4] Particulates were generated by a smoking machine. Figure 8.10 shows the results of these tests

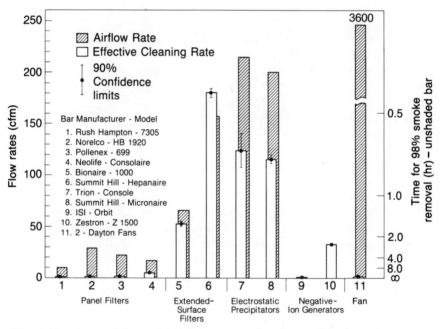

Fig. 8.10. A comparison of the performance of various unducted air-cleaning devices. Shaded bar, airflow rates in cubic feet per minute (cfm); unshaded bar, effective cleaning rates in cfm and the time required for 98 percent smoke removal. The numbered key for each bar gives the manufacturer and model number: 1, Rush Hampton 7305; 2, Norelco HB 1920; 3, Pollenex 699; 4, Neolife Consolaire; 5, Bionaire 1000; 6, Summit Hill Hepanaire; 7, Trion Console; 8, Summit Hill Micronaire; 9, ISI Orbit; 10, Zestron Z 1500; 11, Dayton Fans (2). Source: F. J. Offermann *et al.*, *Control of Respirable Particulates and Radon Progeny with Portable Air Cleaners*, Lawrence Berkeley Laboratory Report LBL-16659 (1983).

for particulates of size 0.45 micrometer. This is approximately the mass median diameter for cigarette smoke particulates; that is, half the particulate mass comes from particles greater than that size and half from smaller particles. The shaded bars show the actual airflow rates through the devices. The unshaded bars show the effective cleaning rates in cubic feet per minute (cfm) and the time required for 98 percent smoke removal in hours (right-hand axis).

The performances of the various devices varied substantially: effective air-cleaning rates ranged from zero for the small fan-filter devices to 180 cfm for the high-efficiency particulate air (HEPA) filter device. The residential negative-ion generator also had an effective air-cleaning rate of zero, even with two large fans to help. The commercial air ionizer had a moderate effect on particulate concentrations, but it had no collector surfaces; thus, the room surfaces became the collecting surfaces.

The two electrostatic precipitators and the two extended-surface filter devices were the most effective devices tested. Extended-surface filters have a larger ratio of filter media area to face area than the small filters; the HEPA filter is a special type of extended-surface filter. The power requirements of these devices are greater than for the other ones. The power demands for these four air cleaners are 32, 67, 109, and 77 watts, respectively, from left to right in the figure.

Very few tests of the effectiveness of electronic air cleaners have been reported in the indoor-air-quality literature. One investigation worth discussing was performed at the John Pierce Foundation in New Haven, Connecticut, by William Cain and Brian Leaderer.[5] The main objective of their experiments was to determine the ventilation requirements in occupied rooms with or without cigarette smokers present. The criteria used to establish ventilation rates were measured levels of carbon monoxide and total suspended particulates (TSP) and odor levels as judged by both smokers and nonsmokers. The smoking took place in an aluminum-lined chamber of 1,200 cubic feet that had an adjustable ventilation system.

TSP, carbon monoxide, and odor levels were monitored for various rates of smoking (4 to 16 cigarettes per hour). The short-term national ambient air quality standard for TSP (260 micrograms per cubic meter for 24 hours) was often exceeded, even at 4 cigarettes per hour and strong ventilation (18 cubic feet per minute per person). Approximately 98 percent of the particulates (by volume) fell between 0.05 and 1.0 micrometer across, all in the respirable range. In the case of particulates generated by cigarettes, as discussed in Chapter 7, many of the particulates are toxic (such as nicotine) and pose a significant health risk if inhaled and deposited in the lungs.

Figure 8.11 shows the change in TSP concentration over time after

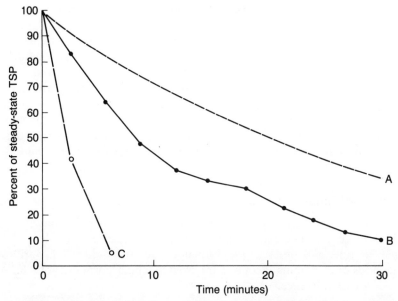

Fig. 8.11. The decay of total suspended particulates (TSP) under three conditions. Curve A is a theoretical curve applicable where particulates are removed by ventilation only. Curve B is the actual decay with a ventilation rate of 44 cubic feet per minute. Curve C shows the decay when recirculated air is passed through an electrostatic precipitator. Source: W. S. Cain and B. P. Leaderer, "Ventilation Requirements in Occupied Spaces During Smoking and Nonsmoking Occupancy," *Environment International*, vol. 8 (1982). Reprinted with permission from Pergamon Press, Ltd., and the author.

smoking stopped and after a steady-state level of TSP was reached. Curve A indicates the decay that would be expected if only a typical ventilation rate of 11 cubic feet per minute per person (44 cfm total) were responsible for TSP removal; curve B shows the actual decay rate of TSP. Curve C shows the decay when the recirculated air was passed through an electrostatic precipitator. The reason curve B is steeper than curve A is that some particulates are adsorbed on surfaces in the chamber, thus increasing the rate of removal over the theoretical rate. Adsorbed particulates, however, carry condensed gaseous materials that cause a lingering odor. Higher ventilation rates or cleaning of the recirculated air may be necessary to overcome this effect.

The rapid decay of TSP when the smoky air is passed through an electrostatic precipitator indicates the effectiveness of these air cleaners. Ninety percent of the total particulate mass is removed in about 5 minutes by the precipitator, whereas ventilation and natural adsorption take at least 30 minutes to achieve the same reduction. There are no data on the ability of electrostatic precipitators to control cigarette smoke particulates while smoking is in progress, but Cain and Leaderer's study suggests that precipitators would be quite effective. A list of manufacturers of residential-sized electronic air cleaners can be found in Appendix B.

In summary, small fan-filter air cleaners are not effective particulate-reduction devices. Some ion generators are moderately effective air cleaners. Both electrostatic precipitators and extended-surface filters (including HEPA filters) are very effective at reducing particulate concentrations. The power demand for the effective air cleaners varies from approximately 50 to 100 watts.

Control of Other Pollutants

It remains to review control techniques for several pollutants previously discussed. These are combustion products (carbon dioxide, nitrogen dioxide, and other gases), formaldehyde, and radon. The various methods of contaminant control are listed in tabular form in Tables 8.1–8.3 for easy reference.

Table 8.1. Techniques for the Control of Combustion Products

Control method	Specific control	Comments
Removal	Separate garage (and associated auto emissions) from house	
Substitution	Replace combustion appliances with electric appliances or solar-heating systems	Capital cost of electric ranges is $220 to $710; gas and electric ranges with comparable features are comparably priced
Change in design	Install pilotless combustion appliances or retrofit appliances with electronic ignition	Pilotless ranges cost $50 more than ranges with pilot lights
Spatial confinement	Place combustion appliances in isolated rooms; oil- and gas-combustion heating units may be placed outside house	
Local ventilation	Use local ventilation for combustion appliances	Capital cost of exhaust fans is $40 to $50; capital cost of range hoods is $85 to $230

SOURCE: *Indoor Air Quality Handbook* (Albuquerque, NM: Sandia National Laboratories and AnaChem, Inc., 1982).

Table 8.2. Techniques for the Control of Formaldehyde

Control method	Specific control	Comments
Change in design	Naturally age particle board and other urea-formaldehyde-containing products or induce aging by heat treatment to cause outgassing before use	Effectiveness unknown
Substitution	Use thermal insulation other than urea-formaldehyde foam	
Substitution	Replace particle board with solid wood	
Encapsulation	Cover particle board with shellac, varnish, polymeric coating, or other diffusion barriers	Effectiveness unknown

SOURCE: *Indoor Air Quality Handbook* (Albuquerque, NM: Sandia National Laboratories and AnaChem, Inc., 1982).

Table 8.3. Techniques for the Control of Radon and Radon Daughters

Control method	Specific control
Removal	Do not build in areas of uranium or phosphate mining or where tailings have been used for landfill
Removal	Excavate high-radium-containing soil and fill with low-radium-containing soil
Substitution	Use building materials with low radium content, not high radium content
Encapsulation	Seal cracks in basement walls and concrete slabs with polymeric caulks to prevent introduction of radon from soil
Encapsulation	Cover basement walls and concrete slabs with epoxy paint, polymeric sealant, or polyethylene or polyamide film (vapor barrier) to prevent introduction of radon from soil or concrete
Encapsulation	Improve slab construction to reduce cracks through which radon can penetrate
Local ventilation	Ventilate crawlspace
Physical filtration	Use high-efficiency particulate air filtration
Electrostatic interaction	Use electrostatic precipitation

SOURCE: *Indoor Air Quality Handbook* (Albuquerque, NM: Sandia National Laboratories and AnaChem, Inc., 1982).

9

Indoor Air Quality Problems in Office Buildings

A few days after moving into a brand-new office building in Port Washington, New York, more than half of almost 200 Itel employees were feeling ill. This mysterious illness consisted of headache, eye irritation, drowsiness, fatigue, nausea, dizziness, and throat irritation. Because of fears that these symptoms might be signs of Legionnaire's disease or some other mysterious ailment, the Itel workers moved into nearby trailers while a team of epidemiologists investigated.[1]

Dozens of workers at a newly refurbished office building in downtown New York City came down with a variety of symptoms upon moving into their new quarters. Employees of NBC and Simon and Schuster reported suffering headaches, skin rashes, breathing difficulties, and fatigue since they moved into the Simon and Schuster building on the Avenue of the Americas.[2] Many of these workers have quit their jobs; others have bought air cleaners at their own expense. Incidents like these have been repeated in hundreds of newly constructed or remodeled office and school buildings throughout the United States and around the world.

NIOSH, the National Institute of Occupational Safety and Health, has investigated complaints in approximately 200 office buildings across the United States.[3] Typical complaints are eye and throat irritation, shortness of breath, headaches, dizziness, chest tightness, and fatigue. In only about one-tenth of these buildings were specific sources of pollution determined to be the cause: some of the sources identified were motor vehicle exhaust from a nearby garage, asphalt fumes from roofing materials, and organic compounds from carpet glue, paints, and solvents. In the vast majority of cases, no specific chemical or biological agent was found in concentrations high enough to cause the illnesses reported. Inadequate ventilation was presumed to be the cause, for in 70 percent of these buildings, the windows were sealed and air was recirculated through a central air-conditioning system. The name *tight-building syndrome* has been coined to designate the combination of symptoms found in these buildings.

Office buildings differ from residential buildings in several important ways. First, in most new office buildings fresh outside air is supplied through mechanical ventilation systems, and little air infiltrates into the building from the outside. Windows are made inoperable in order to tighten the building shell and reduce infiltration. Second, air is recirculated throughout these buildings; a significant fraction of the air brought in from the outside is reused before being exhausted. This is done to reduce the costs of cooling hot outside air in the summer and heating cold outside air in the winter. Both of these factors lead to higher concentrations of indoor-generated contaminants—but, as stated above, in only a few cases do specific air pollutants definitely underlie illnesses.

One of the most difficult problems facing researchers in the indoor air-quality field is determining the causes of office-building sickness. We have clues and partial answers, but in most cases ventilation is the explanation of last resort.

Ventilation Requirements in Nonresidential Buildings

Nonresidential buildings include schools, department stores, offices, and public buildings. Most nonresidential buildings are designed to incorporate ventilation systems that circulate air throughout the building to maintain air temperature and humidity within the comfort range.

In addition to providing heated or cooled air for maintenance of comfort, the system must also provide outside air (also called ventilation air) to occupied spaces. This ventilation of buildings with outside air is required to (1) establish a satisfactory balance between the oxygen and carbon dioxide in the occupied environment, (2) remove moisture from internal sources, (3) dilute odors to an acceptable level, and (4) remove contaminants produced by human activity, building materials, and other sources within the ventilated space.

The American Society of Heating, Refrigeration, and Air Conditioning Engineers (ASHRAE) has developed ventilation standards giving recommended and minimum ventilation rates for many types of building spaces.[4] Although voluntary, these widely accepted standards have been adopted by many states and local governments in their building codes. Prompted by the desire to conserve energy in buildings, in the mid-1970's ASHRAE published a new standard for energy-efficient building design, which recommended that the minimum ventilation rates be used in designs for new buildings. The minimum allowable ventilation rate for occupied spaces is 5.0 cfm (cùbic feet per minute) per person. Thus, an office-building space designed for twenty occupants will require a minimum ventilation rate of 100 cubic feet of outside air every minute. A small fan could move that much air; however, the outside air requirement is usually a small fraction of the total air circulating through an office building. Therefore, large fans capable of moving thousands of cubic feet per minute are required. The total air circulation (outside air plus recirculated air) in office buildings is determined by heating and cooling demands.

The minimum ventilation rate is partially based on the need to dilute the carbon dioxide produced by metabolism and expired from the lungs; 5 cfm per person allows an adequate safety factor to account for health and diet variations and some increased activity levels beyond that of typical sedentary office workers. Symptoms of exposure to high carbon dioxide levels are headaches, deep and rapid breathing, and loss of judgment. The U.S. occupational health standard for carbon dioxide is 5,000 ppm. Removal of indoor-generated moisture is not an important problem because there are usually no significant indoor sources of water vapor other than the occupants themselves. In very humid climates, dehumidifiers may be added to air-conditioning systems.

Ventilation requirements were originally established to keep odors in occupied spaces at an acceptable level. Throughout history, bad-smelling places have been thought of as unhealthy. Over 40 years ago, two researchers at the Harvard School of Public Health undertook one of the most complete studies of odors and ventilation requirements ever performed.[5] They placed sedentary persons in a chamber and had observers enter after several hours and rate the intensity of body odor. They determined how odor in the chamber varied with the density of occupation and with the rate of ventilation. All subjects in these experiments were nonsmokers. The Harvard experiments and the carbon dioxide dilution requirement have been the basis of the ASHRAE ventilation standards until recently, and the standards are only now being updated to consider pollutants other than body odor. Thus, in situations where the major source of pollutants is not the occupants but materials in the building (for example, particle board that emits formaldehyde), the new standards may call for additional ventilation. In the proposed standards, the ventilation requirements for areas where smoking is allowed are about three times greater than for similar nonsmoking areas. Therefore, if the proposed standards are adopted, there will be a quantifiable additional cost of heating, cooling, and moving excess ventilation air in buildings where smoking is allowed.

Pollutant Sources and Health Effects

Most of the sources of indoor air pollution previously discussed can be found in nonresidential as well as residential buildings. Several pollutants that are of great concern in houses, such as radon and combustion products, are rarely found in high concentrations in nonresidential buildings. By contrast, a number of pollutants and environmental factors are of more concern in nonresidential buildings: these include airborne microbes, asbestos, a wide variety of organics, air ions, and lighting quality.

In a number of problem office buildings, measurements have been made of formaldehyde and other organics, carbon dioxide, carbon monoxide, nitrogen dioxide, and particulates. In most cases, each of these contaminants is present at concentrations higher than outdoors but lower than applicable health standards. It is possible that several contaminants acting together, or acting with other environmental factors, cause some of the symptoms seen in these office buildings.

Organic Compounds

Measurements carried out by the Lawrence Berkeley Laboratory in a newly built San Francisco office building are representative of surveys in other office buildings. Table 9.1 summarizes the results of indoor and outdoor measurements and relevant air quality standards for one section of the eight-story office building.[6] Except for carbon dioxide and formaldehyde, the relevant standards were outdoor air quality standards established by the Environmental Protection Agency (see Chapter 1). None of the contaminants measured was found at concentrations greater than the

Table 9.1. Measured Air Pollutant Levels in a San Francisco Office Building and Air Quality Standards

Contaminant	Building air quality		Air quality standards	
	Concentration	Averaging time	Concentration	Averaging time
Carbon monoxide	4 ppm	1 hr	35 ppm	1 hr
Carbon dioxide	1,000 ppm	8 hrs	5,000 ppm	8 hrs
Nitrogen dioxide	30 ppb	1 wk	50 ppb	1 yr
Hydrocarbons	2.5 ppm	30 mins	No standard	
Formaldehyde	0.04 ppm	6 hrs	0.1–0.7 ppm	Maximum
Aldehydes	0.09 ppm	6 hrs	No standard	
Particulates	31 $\mu g/m^3$	12 hrs	75 $\mu g/m^3$	1 yr
			260 $\mu g/m^3$	24 hrs
Lead	0.2 $\mu g/m^3$	12 hrs	1.5 $\mu g/m^3$	3 mos

SOURCE: I. Turiel *et al.*, "The Effects of Reduced Ventilation on Indoor Air Quality in an Office Building," *Atmospheric Environment*, vol. 17, no. 1 (1983).

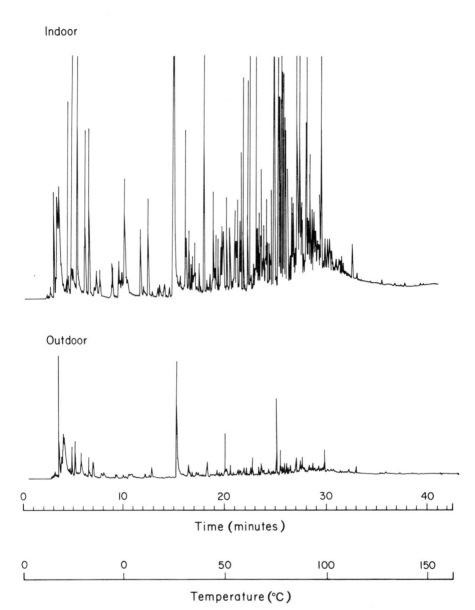

Indoor

Outdoor

Time (minutes)

Temperature (°C)

Fig. 9.1. A comparison of the levels of gaseous organic compounds inside and outside an office building where indoor air quality complaints were registered. Time refers to the gas chromatograph's experimental run (in which temperature is slowly raised), and roughly corresponds to molecular weight. Source: R. R. Miksch *et al.*, "Trace Organic Chemical Contaminants in Office Spaces," *Environment International*, vol. 8 (1982).

relevant standard. More than 40 organic compounds were found in the indoor environment at levels higher than the outdoors. Individual contaminants were all well below workplace standards set by the Occupational Safety and Health Administration, but many of these toxic compounds are not usually present simultaneously in industrial environments where the OSHA standards apply. Many researchers are concerned that a number of these compounds acting together can affect health in building occupants.

Figure 9.1 shows gas chromatograms of organic material found in the indoor and outdoor air for this same San Francisco office building. Organic compounds were greater in number and concentration indoors than outdoors, as indicated by the number and sizes of peaks. The largest peaks fell into one of three classes of compounds: solvents (petroleum distillates) and hydrocarbons derived from them, alkylated aromatic hydrocarbons that are solvents themselves or constituents of solvent mixtures, and chlorinated hydrocarbons. At high concentrations, these compounds are known to cause eye and respiratory irritation, and some (trichloroethylene and benzene) are suspected of being carcinogens. Other

Table 9.2. Organic Compounds Identified in Indoor Air

Compound[a]	Approximate ratio (indoor/outdoor)	Approximate concentration (ppb)
Hydrocarbons		
n-heptane	10	20
n-octane	80	300
n-nonane	100	150
cyclohexane		
hexane		
many other branched aliphatics		
Aromatics		
benzene	5	25
toluene	5	75
xylenes	15	150
trimethylbenzene		
ethylbenzene		
ethylmethylbenzene		
Halogenated compounds		
tetrachloroethylene		large
trichloroethylene		small
1,1,1-trichloroethane		small

SOURCE: C. D. Hollowell and R. R. Miksch, *Sources and Concentrations of Organic Compounds in Indoor Environments*, Lawrence Berkeley Laboratory Report LBL-13195 (July 1981).

[a] Compounds identified were present in air sampled at an LBL office trailer (90 G) and/or a San Francisco office building. Numerical data is for the San Francisco office building only.

researchers have found similar compounds in the air of office buildings. The combined health effect of these organic compounds is unknown but potentially of great concern. Table 9.2 lists some of the organic compounds typically found indoors. Table 2.10 summarizes the health effects of some of these compounds.

Formaldehyde is one organic compound that was measured separately. Its concentration averaged about 30 to 50 percent of the current health standard (0.1 ppm) for the European countries. The concentration of formaldehyde in this building is typical of other office buildings, that is, substantially higher indoors than outdoors but below current applicable health standards.

Gaseous Pollutants

Carbon dioxide concentrations measured in a number of school and office buildings have always been below 5,000 ppm, the occupational standard. As Figure 9.2 illustrates, the concentration of carbon dioxide follows the occupancy pattern, reaching a maximum concentration of almost 1,600 ppm in the afternoon. The measurements were made at breathing height (5 feet above the floor) in a public waiting room in the previously mentioned office building. In buildings where the ventilation is inadequate, carbon dioxide levels could become higher in regions of low air movement than average readings such as these would indicate. A large number of room dividers may also slow the airflow in an office. If carbon dioxide is concentrated by several times in stagnant pockets, some of the symptoms experienced by office workers in poorly ventilated buildings, such as headaches and respiratory difficulties, could be partially caused by carbon dioxide. Whether or not that is the case, high carbon dioxide concentrations can definitely be used as an indicator of poor ventilation.

Carbon monoxide concentrations inside nonresidential buildings rarely exceed the EPA health standards. There are no significant indoor sources of carbon monoxide other than tobacco smoke. There have been cases where high carbon monoxide concentrations were recorded indoors, owing to strong outdoor sources. Heavy traffic and nearby garages emanate carbon monoxide, nitrogen oxides, and odorous gases that may be drawn into the ventilation system. Needless to say, intake vents should be located well above ground and far from any sources of air pollution. It is also prudent to place intake vents a reasonable distance from exhaust vents to prevent exhaust air from being sucked back into the building with the intake air.

Copying machines are potential sources of ozone; some wet-process machines may also be sources of ammonia and organic compounds. Rooms where copiers are located should be well ventilated to prevent

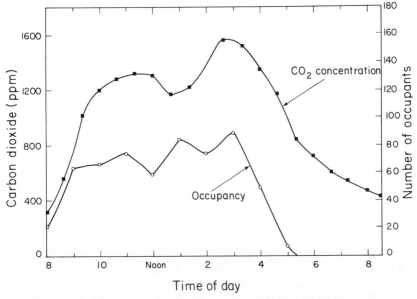

Fig. 9.2. Time dependence of occupancy and of carbon dioxide (CO_2) concentration in the waiting room of a San Francisco office building. The ventilation system is in the recirculation mode. Source: I. Turiel *et al.*, "The Effects of Reduced Ventilation on Indoor Air Quality in an Office Building," *Atmospheric Environment*, vol. 17, no. 1 (January 1983).

buildup of these pollutants. Because of its strong pungent odor, ozone is easily recognizable. Oxygen can be converted into ozone by any source of ultraviolet light or electric discharge. In cities with photochemical smog, the outdoor air brought in through the ventilation system may be a more significant ozone source than copying machines.

Particulates

If gaseous pollutants, even in amounts below the standards, can be counted as factors behind the tight-building syndrome, then neither are particulates above suspicion. Some outbreaks of symptoms have been traced to the residue of carpet shampoos. A more insidious factor is the air ion level inside office buildings. Chapter 4 pointed out that ions are removed from the air by dust particles, which settle on the nearest object, and that in the absence of an ion source, indoor air tends to become depleted of ions. This also holds true for the typical well-sealed, mechanically ventilated office building. The results on health have not been studied thoroughly.

More is known about airborne microbes. Some outbreaks, such as the measles epidemic in the elementary school mentioned in Chapter 4, are straightforward instances of contagious microbes being blown around in a building full of susceptible people. Other more famous cases have been both vexing to researchers and deadly to building occupants. Not least of these is Legionnaire's disease, now known to medicine as legionellosis.

Hypersensitivity Pneumonitis and Humidifier Lung

Microorganisms growing in air-conditioning systems have caused outbreaks of respiratory illness in a number of office buildings. Some of these organisms grow in the water reservoirs of humidifiers or in cooling towers of air-conditioning systems. Some systems use humidifiers to treat incoming air after it is heated and its relative humidity is lowered. A complex mixture of organisms may grow in a water reservoir, including amoebas, bacteria, molds, and fungi.

Twenty-six of 50 office employees of a large factory in Tennessee periodically experienced flu-like symptoms (fever, chills, headaches, chest tightness, and breathing difficulty) on Monday nights after returning home from work.[7] Their symptoms usually subsided by the next morning and did not return until the following Monday evening. Only employees working in a section of the factory served by one particular heating and cooling unit that used a humidifier were afflicted. Removing the humidification system eliminated the symptoms, and no cases of the "Monday miseries" have been reported since. Epidemiologists from the University of Tennessee came to the conclusion that an allergic reaction to microorganisms growing in the humidifier reservoir caused the respiratory illness. The specific organism responsible for the allergic reaction (known as humidifier lung) was not identified, although they suspect it was an amoeba.

Hypersensitivity pneumonitis is a similar disease but more serious in its health effects. In this disease, inflammation in the alveolar walls and peripheral bronchioles results from an allergic reaction to inhaled organisms. Repeated or continuous exposure to the allergen may lead to pulmonary fibrosis. The suspected organism causing this disease is a heat-resistant fungus. It has been found in humidifier fluid, air conditioners, and evaporative coolers.

Legionnaire's Disease

An outbreak of pneumonia among several thousand persons attending a 1976 American Legion convention in Philadelphia's Bellevue Stratford Hotel resulted in 182 illnesses and 29 deaths.[8] The bacterium causing the disease, *Legionella*, was previously unrecognized and appeared to have spread among the victims by an airborne route.

It took 2 years to isolate the probable cause of the pneumonia. After a number of potential agents of disease were considered, such as nickel carbonyl poisoning, swine influenza, and food poisoning, it was concluded that the bacteria came from water in the air-conditioning system. In this first outbreak, and in a number of other cases of legionellosis, soil excavation took place at the time of outbreaks, and it is thought that the bacteria were released from the soil into the air. Interestingly, health surveys have shown that a large percentage of healthy people carry antibodies to *Legionella*; this implies that exposure to it is common and that infection is also common, though not always recognized.

James Imperato, of the State University of New York Medical Center in Brooklyn, studied nine outbreaks of legionellosis throughout the world.[9] He identified two distinct but clinically related illnesses caused by the bacterium, a severe and fatal version and a mild version. Imperato stated, "Reported epidemics and sporadic cases probably represent only a small portion of the actual incidence of the disease. As with many other diseases, epidemics are discovered when an inquisitive individual searches for them or when their explosive nature draws attention."

Chemicals are often used to kill microorganisms that can live in air-conditioning systems. However, periodic treatment is necessary, since otherwise the microorganisms can quickly recolonize. A better control technique is to design air-conditioning systems that do not allow microorganisms to survive and multiply. One potentially effective technique is to vary the temperature of water reservoirs to create an unfavorable environment for microorganisms. Additional research is needed to evaluate such strategies.

Carpet Shampoos

Outbreaks of respiratory and eye irritation have been shown to be caused by detergent residues left in carpets after shampooing. The symptoms include coughing and dry throat and are usually localized to a specific area of the building. The National Institute of Occupational Safety and Health (NIOSH) has investigated several buildings where respiratory and eye irritation have occurred.

In one city government building, 30 of 45 employees complained of one or more respiratory tract symptoms.[10] They had high rates of cough, dry throat, difficulty in breathing, nasal congestion, and headaches. It took several months before the employees realized that pounding or scuffing the carpet released a substance that was irritating when inhaled. Some employees recalled that their symptoms began shortly after the city had bought a carpet shampoo machine. The shampoo product had been improperly diluted, resulting in a solution several times more concentrated than what the manufacturer recommended. Areas with heavy traffic were shampooed most frequently, and workers in these areas had the highest rates of respiratory irritation. Their symptoms disappeared when the chemical residue was removed from the carpets.

All ten staff members of a day-care center and most of the children developed respiratory irritation after returning from a spring vacation.[11] The carpet, shampooed during the spring break, was the cause. It took three washings to remove the residue left on the carpet and to end symptoms in the children and teachers.

Another instance (although not in office buildings) may point to factors other than shampoo. Researchers studying an outbreak of 23 cases of Kawasaki syndrome in eastern Colorado homes in the spring of 1982 found an association between the application of rug shampoo and the syndrome in children under 5.[12] Kawasaki syndrome is an acute illness characterized by fever, rash, and fissured lips. Serious complications can occur, such as inflammation and widening of the coronary and other arteries, which in turn may lead to blood clots or the rupture of blood vessels. The researchers hypothesized that some infectious or allergenic agent in the carpets had been disturbed during the cleaning procedure and become airborne. They did not think that detergents left over from the shampooing could have caused the type of illness that they observed. Thus, it appears that the shampooing of carpets may cause illness in two different ways: first, by the inhalation of detergent residue; and second, by the inhalation of infectious or allergenic agents made airborne by the process of shampooing.

Psychophysiological Factors

In most cases of tight-building syndrome, specific chemical or microbial causes were not identified. This has sometimes led building managers and others to suggest that the illnesses were psychologically based and not a result of poor indoor air quality. It is difficult to estimate the relative importance of direct physical effects from air pollutants and the overall impact of the working environment. For instance, there are numerous causes of stress on an office worker, such as noise, tight deadlines, crowding, and air pollutants. According to present theories of stress, chemical, physical, and psychological agents all act on an individual to produce stress. The sum of the individual effects of these agents may be enough to cause adverse health effects.

A few of these agents—air ions, lighting, and video display terminals

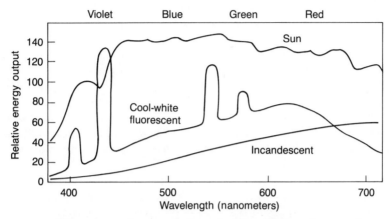

Fig. 9.3. The spectral outputs of a standard incandescent lamp and a cool-white fluorescent lamp are shown relative to the solar spectrum.

(VDT's)—have aroused attention and even controversy. Air ions (see Chapter 4) appear to affect mood as well as causing physical symptoms, and sensitive persons may be adversely affected by ion-scarce office environments. Although lighting and VDT's are not indoor air contaminant sources, they are discussed briefly because of their potential importance as stressors leading to tight-building syndrome.

Most offices use fluorescent lighting. The standard "cool white" fluorescent lamp has a spectral output that is significantly different from that of sunlight (see Fig. 9.3). Research is under way in many laboratories to determine whether light from fluorescent lamps has adverse biological effects on humans. An Australian study found an association between malignant melanoma (skin cancer) and exposure to fluorescent lighting at work.[13] Additional investigations are necessary to establish radiation from fluorescent lights as the causative agent.

Older (pre-1978) fluorescent fixtures contain in their ballasts polychlorinated biphenyls (PCB's), suspected carcinogens. PCB's may be released as a vapor when these older lamps catch fire or explode. Fluorescent lamps are also subject to fixture hum and flicker, both of which may produce stress. Inadequate lighting levels may also produce stress in building occupants.

VDT's are another potential source of stress in the work environment. Several sensational stories in the media have reported on unexpectedly high rates of miscarriages and birth defects among pregnant VDT operators.[14] Typical complaints include headaches, eyestrain, and other visual and musculoskeletal problems. Canadian and American studies of VDT's have found no indication that radiation emissions are intense enough to cause any health problems.[15] There is certain to be additional research on the health effects of VDT use.

Workers who feel somewhat ill but cannot identify the source of their illness may be susceptible to suggestions concerning potential causes of their illness. The sudden presence of an unusual, unpleasant odor could prompt these people to lay the blame for their illnesses on this known annoyance. The number of workers reporting symptoms may increase as the notion of the source of illness spreads. This mass expression of illness is called mass psychogenic illness by health professionals (and mass hysteria by headline writers).

A few suspected cases of mass illness have been reported. Half of the employees at a newly constructed state archives building in Tallahassee, Florida, experienced headaches and symptoms of upper respiratory tract irritation. Symptoms usually began within 30 minutes of entering the building each morning and disappeared on weekends and holidays. Several physicians and epidemiologists from NIOSH and other government agencies investigated this "mysterious malady," as the press called it.[16] All employees were asked to fill out a report whenever they felt ill.

Extensive environmental monitoring furnished no clues; doctors who examined symptomatic employees found no objective clinical or laboratory abnormalities. The epidemiologists suggested, in their report to the director of the Centers for Disease Control, that a psychogenic cause was possible. Another possibility was that regardless of the initiating event (a toxic gas or viral illness, perhaps), the illnesses were perpetuated by wide publicity, the naming of the illness, the log kept for each victim, and the change from a passive reporting system to a more active recruitment system when reports of illness decreased. It was also noted that "previous analyses of mass illness indicated that such illness is usually caused by the combination of certain personality traits with a stressful, unpleasant, and often poorly managed work environment."

Another incident of mass illness in a building occurred in a university data-processing center where 35 keypunch operators suddenly had symptoms of fainting, dizziness, and nausea after complaining of a strange odor.[17] Monitoring the indoor air quality and medical exams did not detect any causative agents in the building. When they were told that their illness was probably caused by a combination of transient atmospheric conditions that had now passed on, the keypunch operators returned to work with no further outbreaks.

Michael Colligan of NIOSH has discussed two ways in which indoor air quality may psychologically affect building occupants.[18] The first involves direct effects in an individual on such response symptoms as information processing, sensorimotor performance, and learning. The second involves the overall impact of the environment on the autonomic (self-controlling) nervous system. Colligan stated, "Air quality is one of many possible sources of stress that challenge the organism. . . . The impact of nontoxic but aversive properties of various chemicals on an individual's level of general arousal, perceived threat, and anxiety have yet to be defined."

Most investigators of mass illness in buildings agree that it is important for management to take the complaints of employees seriously. Employees should be encouraged to communicate among themselves and with management. In California, workers who had contact with the chemical dibromochloropropane discovered, through casual conversations with coworkers, that many of them were unable to father children, a discovery that led to regulations on the use of this chemical. Even though outbreaks of mass illness may occasionally be perpetuated by employee activism, there are very likely underlying physiological causes of the initial illness. Enlightened managers can benefit both employees and the company by cooperating in the process of uncovering the causes of mass illness.

Improving Office Air

Some of the human factors behind tight-building syndrome are approachable through better business management, most notably those factors related to workplace stress. But whatever a manager's response is to an outbreak of symptoms, there is no substitute for a thorough check of the building itself. Some measures can be taken only when a new building is designed; others are suitable for existing buildings.

Ventilation Systems

The air in most problem office buildings can be made more healthful and comfortable by increasing the amount of ventilation air brought inside to dilute indoor-generated air pollutants. There are some exceptions, for example, when the intake vents are located at street level near heavy traffic. Unfortunately, there is a significant expense associated with heating or cooling this extra outside air during much of the year; however, this expense may be offset by the higher productivity brought about by a healthier working environment.

More research is needed on how effectively ventilation systems distribute air throughout the occupied spaces in a building. Ventilation rates are usually measured, if they are measured at all, in large central air ducts and not in the localized space of an office worker, where partitions and other factors may significantly lower local ventilation rates. In one San

Francisco office building, 25 percent less ventilation air reached the offices on the first floor than air-duct measurements suggested.[19] If ventilation air quantities could be measured in an occupant's breathing space, even greater deficiencies might be evident. Accurate portable measuring devices are not yet made to perform such a study.

In the same office building, many instances were found of ventilation air short-circuiting as it entered an office space. Fresh air entering a space from a ceiling air diffuser was found to be moving directly to a nearby exhaust vent and not reaching the workers. This short-circuiting of ventilation air is not uncommon and may result when supply air velocity is low and when the supply and exhaust vents are improperly placed relative to each other.

Two other reasons ventilation systems may not perform as designed are defective equipment and improper installation or poor placement of intake vents. Cases have been reported where intake vents were located near exhaust vents, or near other sources of air pollution such as underground garages or garbage receptacles. A brand-new state office building in Sacramento, California, was found, after many employee complaints, to have problems with its ventilation system.[20] Eighty percent of the variable air-volume boxes, which control the fraction of air recirculated, were defective. Some of the main air-supply fans had defective controller cables, making them operate at reduced capacity. Finally, many of the supply vents into the office areas had not even been opened to let air into the room!

Many of these problems can be solved by testing ventilation systems thoroughly before buildings are occupied. Sensitivity to employee complaints should also serve management in uncovering problems associated with the working environment.

Building Materials

Careful selection of building materials can reduce the quantity of indoor-generated air pollutants. Particle board and other products containing urea-formaldehyde should be used only where substitutes cannot be found. Furniture, carpets, space partitions, and wall coverings should be chosen to minimize the amount of formaldehyde and other organic gases emitted in the office environment. For example, one study of the organic contaminants emitted from five different samples of carpet material found a wide variation in the type of organics emitted.[21] The least hazardous emanation was from a synthetic-fiber carpet with thin composition backing.

Much research remains to be performed before a catalog of building materials and furnishings and the contaminants they emit can be assembled. In the meantime, some knowledge of particularly hazardous materials is available. It may be cost-effective in the long run to ventilate new office buildings for up to several months before they are occupied. This would allow time for ventilation and indoor air quality tests throughout the building and for the outgassing of contaminants. The ventilation system could be run without any heating or cooling, to save energy; running it with all outside air and no recirculation would allow for rapid disposal of indoor-generated pollutants. There is a timing problem associated with this strategy, for ideally the ventilation should be done after carpets and other furnishings have been installed; but who would pay the rent while the building is unoccupied but leased and furnished? Again, the expense of ensuring adequate indoor air quality may be less than the costs of increased absenteeism and lowered productivity resulting from poor working conditions.

Reduction of Passive Smoking

As was mentioned in Chapter 6, many companies are encouraging their employees to quit smoking. Some employers have actually forbidden employees to smoke while on company property. For the majority of office buildings, where smoking is allowed, some companies are attempting to separate smokers from nonsmokers. Recently, an office worker for the Federal Defense Logistics Agency won a decision in the Ninth U.S. Circuit Court of Appeals in San Francisco entitling her to a smoke-free environment at her place of work.[22] She reacted to cigarette smoke with symptoms of severe bronchitis. The ruling is considered a landmark for workers allergic to smoke and workers with small-airways disease induced by smoke. If the government cannot find a smoke-free workplace environment for such people, these employees may qualify for disability payments. This decision may have far-reaching consequences in all office environments. Separation of smokers from nonsmokers should reduce smoking-related worker complaints in offices. However, much depends upon the fraction of air recirculated from smoking to nonsmoking areas. Ideally, separate ventilation systems should be used for smoking and nonsmoking areas, but present office buildings are generally not designed to allow for that strategy.

Cleaning Products

There are two ways to minimize the adverse effects of cleaning products used in offices. First, cleaning could be done at the end of the work day; by the time work begins again the next morning, the concentration of contaminants will have significantly decreased. This strategy works well for episodic releases of pollutants where the emission occurs over a very short interval. It would not be useful for situations where cleaning materials emanate pollutants at a slowly decreasing rate for days. The second safety measure is to select cleaning products that contain few or no harmful chemicals. It is also important that cleaning personnel use the proper dilutions of rug shampoo and other products.

What Workers Can Do

Occupants of problem office buildings can do much to correct hazardous conditions in their place of work. If they suspect that some factor at work is making them sick, they should record information about their illness. What are the symptoms and when and where do they occur? Are they sick on Mondays only or do the symptoms appear at work each day and disappear at home? A doctor should be seen if necessary. It is important to know if other building occupants have the same or similar symptoms, and to note their locations in the building. It is also worthwhile to document any changes in the building environment that could have precipitated the illness. For example, extensive remodeling that includes new carpets or new furniture (containing urea-formaldehyde) could add significantly to the burden of air contaminants. Increased recycling of air to reduce air-conditioning costs could also increase the concentrations of indoor-generated contaminants. As discussed earlier, installation of word-processing equipment and increased use of VDT's could increase employee stress and make them more vulnerable to the physiological stresses of indoor air pollutants.

After data on employee illnesses have been prepared, the management should be approached. The concerns of the affected employees should be heard by management and a possible cause of the illness sought. If no cause is found, then a representative of management or of the workers (a union official or otherwise) can contact a public health official to initiate a comprehensive investigation. Implicit in this discussion is the assumption that the illnesses are not acute and do not require immediate attention. Serious illnesses may call for a lawyer as well as a doctor (see Chapter 10).

There are a number of governmental agencies that have jurisdiction over health and safety in the workplace. The U.S. Occupational Safety and Health Administration (OSHA) was created in 1970. Federal law states that each employer shall furnish and maintain a workplace free from recognized hazards that are causing or likely to cause serious physical harm. There are branch offices of OSHA throughout the ten federal regions of the United States; their locations and phone numbers are listed in Appendix C. OSHA complaint forms can be obtained by writing or calling one of these offices. The National Institute of Occupational Safety and Health (NIOSH) performs research on the possible causes of illness in buildings but is not responsible for enforcing federal regulations, as is OSHA. One of the situations in which NIOSH performs epidemiological surveys is when initial OSHA investigations do not find an agent that caused the illness in question. NIOSH has performed over 200 indoor air quality investigations in U.S. office buildings.

Twenty-four states have plans that were approved by the federal government for enforcing OSHA regulations. Building occupants located in one of these states (listed in Appendix C) should contact the state office for assistance rather than the federal OSHA office. State plans developed for the private sector must, to the extent permitted by state law, provide coverage for public employees. In Connecticut, state and local government workers are under state jurisdiction, whereas private employees remain under federal jurisdiction.

The investigation of tight-building syndrome continues in this and other nations. Within a few years, enough data should be gathered to enable architects and engineers to design buildings that are healthy to work in. Meanwhile, the immediate solution to many of the current episodes of illness is to adjust malfunctioning ventilation systems.

10

Legal and Regulatory Issues

People who have been made ill by poor air quality inside their homes or offices will generally try to remedy the offending condition themselves, instead of resorting to litigation for recovery of damages. However, where their illnesses have been serious and prolonged, or where fixing the situation is likely to be expensive and difficult, people have sued the manufacturers, distributors, and sellers of the house or building materials that caused the illness. For example, there have recently been a number of lawsuits from homeowners in many states—including Maine, New York, Illinois, Connecticut, Oregon, West Virginia, and Minnesota—for damages arising from urea-formaldehyde foam insulation; some of these lawsuits have been class-action suits.[1] Outcomes have ranged from removal and replacement of the insulation to money awards to compensate for asthma and chronic respiratory diseases. People have also sued employers who have allowed unhealthy conditions to remain after being notified of them.[2]

There are two main types of legal action that will be considered here. The first is private use of the courts to redress the damages caused by indoor contaminants. The second is governmental regulation of the sale of contaminating building materials, as well as government enforcement of indoor air quality standards. There is very little of the second type of regulation at present.

Generally, when adverse health effects have been caused by poor indoor air quality within the home, those affected have sued the manufacturer of the contaminating building materials. If the building materials are part of the structure of the house and cannot be removed without considerable expense and inconvenience, the homeowner may seek redress from the seller, the architect, the contractor, and the builder of the house. Court actions have been based on one or more of the following legal grounds: negligence, strict liability in tort, misrepresentation or fraud, or breach of express or implied warranty.

Legal language is both ponderous and precise, which may make parts of this chapter hard reading. For sound advice on any of the theories or themes expounded here, a law text or an attorney with a gift for explanation is where to go.

Negligence and Strict Liability

A lawsuit based on negligence will require that the plaintiff or injured person prove to the court that the defendant failed to observe the level of care required of a reasonable person or company undertaking a similar activity, such as manufacturing or selling a similar product. Until recent years, when many states adopted the theory of strict liability, a person who became sick from using a certain product had to show some kind of negligence in the manufacture or sale of that product. Because the processes of manufacture are hard to uncover for one who is not privy to industry secrets, and because it may not be easy to pinpoint the exact carelessness of which the defendant was guilty, it was often difficult for a plaintiff who was injured or made sick by a product to recover damages.

Moreover, companies were frequently shielded from negligence suits if all companies had used the same processes of design and manufacture. It was only when some aspect, such as a company's testing process, fell below the industry standard that suits based on negligence might be successful.

More recently, many states such as New York and California have adopted a strict liability theory of product liability. Under this theory, a plaintiff may recover damages from a manufacturer or supplier of an injury-producing product if that product is found to be "defective" (and, in some jurisdictions, unreasonably dangerous), thereby causing injury. Using this basis for a lawsuit eliminates the necessity of locating the negligence in the manufacturing or distribution process, and allows the court to focus on the product. Under this theory of strict liability, people have recovered damages for injuries from asbestos and from formaldehyde in home furnishings.

For example, in a case recently tried in Alaska, Mr. and Mrs. Heritage sought damages against the retailer and manufacturer of their mobile home, claiming that formaldehyde fumes caused painful and disabling lung damage.[3] The trial court ruled in favor of the defendants, and the Heritages appealed to the Alaska Supreme Court. The Supreme Court reversed the trial court's ruling and ordered a new trial. In its decision, the Supreme Court approved a jury instruction requiring the jury to balance the usefulness of the product against the risk of injury inherent in its use. In the Heritage case, as in all strict liability cases, the jury was required to assess whether the known or knowable dangers inherent in the product (formaldehyde) outweighed its utility (as a building material).

Because disagreement exists about the health effects of these materials, expert witnesses may present different conclusions in their testimony. For example, an expert witness in the Heritage case testified that there was no scientific evidence that concentrations of formaldehyde such as were found in the Heritages' mobile home would cause lung damage. This difficulty might arise in any case in which plaintiffs have claimed illness from indoor air pollution, since the causal relationship between the "defective" substance and the harm must be clear and unequivocal even under strict liability theory. As noted earlier, the link is not clearly defined between certain illnesses and exposure to certain indoor air pollutants such as combustion products or formaldehyde.

Implied Warranty of Fitness for Habitation

Other obstacles that plaintiffs must overcome to win lawsuits for injuries caused by poor indoor air quality are based on some lingering legal anachronisms. One of these rules has prohibited any but the original owner of a house or mobile home from suing the original seller or builder for breach of the implied warranty of fitness for habitation. The reason behind this rule prohibiting suits by subsequent owners is that a warranty of fitness is an implied part of many contracts for sale. Because the subsequent owners of a home are not in "privity" of contract with the builder-vendor (that is, they did not enter directly into a contract of sale with the original builder or seller), subsequent owners were not permitted to sue.

This privity rule has been increasingly overruled throughout the country by courts holding that the implied warranty of fitness extends not only to the first owner, but to subsequent purchasers as well.[4] A suit will generally be permitted for subsequent owners as long as (1) there has not been an unreasonably long lapse of time between the purchase by the first owner and the injury of the subsequent owner; (2) the defects are latent and not easily discoverable by the subsequent purchaser; and (3) there is no great change or alteration in the condition of the house after the original sale.

Use of Contract and Tort Theories

As long as injured people could sue under a strict products liability theory (which is a tort theory, one based on wrongdoing of a noncriminal nature), there would be no need for them to turn to such contractual the-

ories as breach of implied warranty with its attendant privity requirements. However, there are a number of reasons to base lawsuits on breach
of implied warranty as well as on strict product liability. First, it is often
good strategy to allege as many causes of action as are applicable, so that
when all of the evidence is discovered, the groundwork will have been
laid to choose the strongest theory. Therefore, implied warranty, strict
products liability, and negligence often are combined as "counts" of a
single complaint or petition to the court.

Second, the statute of limitations for a tort claim such as strict products liability is commonly shorter than that for a contract claim. Therefore, when people might be too late to sue in tort because too much time
has elapsed from the time the damage was done, they may still have another few years in which to bring a contract suit.

Finally, under the laws of many states, a house itself is not considered
a "product," and thus a suit for breach of contract, rather than one for a
defective product (or even one for the implied warranty of fitness of a
product), is more appropriate. Until the mid-1960's, different rules applied to defects in buildings and defects in products. Where an injured
person might have recovered damages for a foreign object in a soda bottle
or for a lawnmower that ran over its operator when it was supposed to be
in neutral, someone whose house made him or her sick could not recover
damages because of the doctrine of caveat emptor (let the buyer beware).
The main reasons for this doctrine had been that (1) home buyers have
less need of legal protection than buyers of ordinary products because
they have an opportunity to inspect the property they are buying; and (2)
sellers would be subject to unfair penalties if they were subject to claims
for such hidden defects as dry rot, termite damage, soil erosion, or other
conditions that were seen to be beyond their control.

Nevertheless, beginning with mass-produced homes and extending to
real estate in general, in many jurisdictions the rule of caveat emptor as
applied to buildings is gradually eroding. In a number of states, plaintiffs
may now sue the builder-vendors both for implied warranty of fitness for
habitation and for a defective building. Recently, in *Blagg* v. *Fred Hunt
Co., Inc.*, the Supreme Court of Arkansas ruled that the home of the
plaintiffs was a product for the purposes of applying the principles of
strict products liability. This allowed the plaintiffs to recover damages
suffered from formaldehyde fumes and odors that were traced to the carpet and carpet pad installed by the builder.

Recovery in a lawsuit for adverse health effects due to poor indoor air
quality is not always based on a product's being defective as it stands. A
product may be potentially safe and nonpolluting, but the defect arises
from poor assembly instructions (if the user is to be the one assembling

it) or inadequate warnings about safe use of the product. As mentioned earlier, if a defect is not scientifically known or knowable at the time of manufacture or sale, or if the danger in the product's use is outweighed by its usefulness or by the great potential cost that would be involved in making it less dangerous, a court might well rule that a product is not defective.

Perhaps the most active area of litigation has been based on the use of formaldehyde in urea-formaldehyde foam insulation and particle board.

During the 1970's and early 1980's, over 500,000 homes in the United States and 100,000 homes in Canada were retrofit with UF foam insulation in order to reduce their energy use and to lower heating bills. The governments of both nations encouraged such retrofits by offering tax credits. During the last 3 years, over 2,000 individual lawsuits alleging personal injury from formaldehyde exposure have been filed in the United States. In Quebec alone, there are over 2,500 pending lawsuits concerned with UF foam insulation.[5] The Canadian government has decided to give all homeowners of homes in which UF foam was installed $5,000 to defray the cost of removal, which has been estimated at about $10,000.

A single law firm in Buffalo has filed class actions on behalf of all residents within six states (Connecticut, Illinois, Maine, New York, Oregon, and West Virginia) who have UF foam insulation in their homes. To date, none of the courts have decided their class-action certification motions. The New York class-action suit alone, which is against all New York State UF foam installers and their suppliers, totals $2 billion in claims for the approximately 100,000 state residents who bought the product.

Thousands of individual lawsuits have also been filed; a few have been settled before jury decisions and a few others have come to trial. Settlements have ranged from a few thousand dollars to $300,000 in individual actions in site-built residences. One multi-plaintiff settlement directed the developer of 44 new homes to pay the cost of removing and replacing the foam insulation in all homes.[6] Most filed complaints seek compensatory and punitive damages resulting from warranty breaches, negligence, and failure to warn. Jurors interviewed after verdicts have indicated that the defendant's knowledge and its failure to warn was one of the most important factors in their deliberations. In recent cases, juries have also granted awards to occupants of residences where formaldehyde was emitted from particle board in construction materials.

A Rochester, Wisconsin, relocation consultant surveyed 98 real estate appraisers and found that home values decreased 5 to 40 percent (average 14 percent) because of the presence of UF foam insulation.[7] The appraisers said that they base the discount on the cost of removing the insulation. However, once potential buyers know of the presence of the insulation they are often reluctant to purchase the house even with a discount. In Canada, real estate brokers must let potential buyers know of the presence of UF foam insulation in homes listed for sale. In this country, the real estate industry has offered to study such a disclosure plan.[8]

A serious problem related to all these lawsuits is the question of where the money will come from to pay all the claims. At most, only three of the sixteen companies producing the insulation in 1981 are still in business.[9] Many of the remaining companies are in bankruptcy, and their insurance coverage may not be enough to cover all the claims.

Plywood and especially particle board are used extensively in the construction of mobile homes. Both contain formaldehyde, which may be released into the indoor air. As manufacturers of mobile homes have built them "tighter" in response to rising energy prices, complaints from occupants have grown. Owners of mobile homes have successfully brought actions against manufacturers to compensate them for loss of value to the unit and for physical harms resulting from exposure.

Plaintiffs who have successfully proved that formaldehyde exposure damaged their health or significantly reduced the value of their mobile home have been able to seek compensation for both types of harm. Recovery for physical harm tends to be far greater than that for diminished value of the mobile home, owing to the relatively low cost of the units. In 1981, a jury in Washington State awarded $566,000 to a woman who had developed chronic asthma after breathing formaldehyde fumes for only 8 weeks in her new mobile home. Other cases have brought jury awards ranging from $50,000 to $600,000.[10]

Smoking and the Law

Besides bringing suit over indoor air pollution caused by building materials, people have also sought recovery for illness and injury arising from having to work in a smoke-filled environment. However, as with suits for strict products liability for latent defects in houses, the concept of a smoke-free environment is relatively new.

Except for a period in the early 1900's when a number of states forbade the use of cigarettes on moral grounds, there were few or no restrictions on smoking from the 1920's until 1964, the year of the Surgeon General's first report linking lung cancer and smoking. During those years, smoking was the norm and a nonsmoker was often considered to be unusual. Gracious hosts placed cigarettes on their coffee tables for their guests to smoke, and were sure to provide ashtrays everywhere a guest might go.

Today it is a far different world. Increasingly, peer pressure is placed on smokers to refrain; many homeowners and businesses request that people not smoke indoors. State statutes and local ordinances have been enacted to protect people from having to breathe smoke-filled air. Many office managers forbid smoking in workplaces or insist that it be confined to certain nonpublic areas.

These restrictions have come about slowly. Since the time of the Surgeon General's report, there has been a gradual shift in the public's view of smoking. Initially, it was felt that smoking was a self-destructive act but that the nonsmoker had no right to force someone to stop smoking in his or her presence. In the 1970's, however, the danger of sidestream smoke became known, and the concept of the nonsmoker's rights was born.

To date, more than 30 states have legislation prohibiting or restricting smoking in various public places.[11] Such public places include retail stores, restaurants, buses, elevators, museums, concert halls, hospitals, offices, and schools. In addition, many city ordinances prohibit smoking in public places, even where there is no state statute, as do federal agency regulations and private company policies. The public policies behind such statutes and ordinances include fire safety and protection of food, as well as the health protection of nonsmokers.

Nonsmokers who must work in offices with smokers and who do not have company rules to protect them from sidestream smoke may have public-health laws, labor laws, or common-law tort actions to protect them. For example, in the case of *Shimp* v. *Bell Telephone Company*,[12] Shimp had been a receptionist for Bell Telephone for a number of years when she started having nose and eye irritation, constant sore throats, headaches, nausea, and vomiting as a result of her allergy to cigarette smoke. A great number of her coworkers smoked. When she complained, the company did not restrict smoking as it had done in other areas of the office in order to protect sensitive machines. Instead, the company offered to move her to a different location, which would have involved a demotion. It also tried to solve the problem by installing an exhaust fan, which proved ineffective.

The court held that Bell Telephone and employers in general have a duty to provide employees with a reasonably safe workplace. Such a duty would require the employer to ban smoking if the burden on the employer of making and enforcing this prohibition is not unduly great and if the employee cannot find other ways of avoiding the harm. In the Shimp case, the court found that the burden on the employer of prohibiting smoking was not onerous; in fact, Bell Telephone had already banned smoking around certain machines. The court also found that the plaintiff had no way of avoiding the smoke, since she was a receptionist and needed to stay seated in one place most of the time.

The court therefore issued an injunction requiring Bell to provide its employees with a smoke-free workplace. In so doing, legal history was made; the court held that sidestream smoke was indeed toxic to a significant percentage of the population and also that adverse reactions such as those suffered by the plaintiff in the Shimp case were foreseeable.

Nonsmoking employees are increasingly making use of labor laws, public health and occupational safety regulations, and such tort theories as battery or nuisance to stop or recover damages from workplace smoke. Recently the Ninth U.S. Circuit Court of Appeals ruled that Irene Parodi, a federal worker who had a cough and pains in her chest and had experienced trouble breathing for many years, was entitled to a smoke-free workplace.[13] Parodi had filed for disability payments after doctors determined that her sensitivity to cigarette smoke was causing her illness and that her symptoms disappeared when she did not go to work. The court held that she was entitled to receive disability if a smoke-free workplace could not be found for her.

Regulating Indoor Air Pollution

There are no federal indoor air quality regulations that are applicable to residential or commercial buildings; it is far from unanimous that such regulations would be feasible or desirable. In the remainder of this chapter we will consider (1) the ways existing regulatory powers may be used to protect the public health and (2) what additional powers or strategies would be needed to cope with indoor air quality problems.

Precedent exists for government intervention to protect the public health and welfare. The Clean Air Act (discussed in Chapter 1) gives the Environmental Protection Agency authority to regulate certain air pollutants found in the ambient air. The EPA has taken ambient air to mean air outside buildings and decided that it has no power to regulate indoor air quality. The argument can be made that regulation of the ambient air is necessary for the public good, since otherwise there are no incentives for polluters to control their emissions into the outside air. There are at least three types of indoor environments—residential, institutional, and commercial—that must be separately considered when applying such arguments to the indoor air.

Residential Buildings

There is little reason to regulate the quality of indoor air in homes to protect the public good. Residents can decide for themselves whether to safeguard their own indoor air quality. People do not spend much of their time in other people's houses and are therefore not subject to a significant exposure to air contaminants in homes other than their own. Furthermore, homeowners can use some of the control techniques discussed in Chapter 8 and elsewhere in this book.

A counterargument is that individual consumers don't have adequate information on which to base rational decisions concerning appliance or air-cleaner purchases, choice of weatherization measures, and so on. Also, renters do not have full control over their environment when indoors. The role of government, the argument goes, should be to fund research on indoor air quality and make the results of such research public. It is important that some of the publications be written in a format that is understandable to the average person.

Some countries have established ventilation standards for buildings. The idea is that if a specified amount of air exchange takes place, then in general, air pollutant concentrations will be at acceptable levels. The problem with this approach is that strong sources of indoor air pollutants can overwhelm the best ventilation.

In Sweden mechanical ventilation is now required for new homes because they are built very tightly (infiltration rates as low as 0.1 air change per hour). After much study, the Swedish government concluded that there would be too high a probability of indoor air pollutants reaching unhealthy levels unless fans were used to increase the rate of infiltration. Most new homes employ heat exchangers to recover some of the heat that would be otherwise exhausted to the outside (see Chapter 8). The Swedish ventilation standard requires 0.5 air change per hour for residential buildings.

Another approach would be to establish maximum permissible concentrations for various air pollutants in residences. There are at least two problems with this approach. One is the lack of knowledge of all pollutants found in the indoor air. The second problem is that enforcement would be virtually impossible in a nation with 85 million households. Measurement of pollutant levels in millions of homes would cost billions of dollars and would provide information only for the particular time at which the measurements were taken.

Commercial and Institutional Buildings

Public buildings (offices, schools, retail shops) are another matter. In such buildings, individuals do not have the ability to control their environment easily and they rely upon the building manager to provide adequate ventilation air, lighting, and temperature control. Local or state building codes usually have sections dealing with minimum ventilation requirements. As discussed earlier (Chapter 9), these standards are typically identical to the recommendations of the American Society of Heating, Refrigeration, and Air Conditioning Engineers. Air quality is usually acceptable if these regulations are followed in commercial buildings. Most office buildings with indoor air quality problems were found to have improperly installed or defective ventilation equipment.

There are cases of "sick" office buildings where ventilation was according to code and air quality problems were still present. What can be done to prevent such problems from arising in the future? All the answers are not known as yet. Judicious choice of building materials will help; careful maintenance of ventilation and humidifying equipment is also important. Most cities have a system whereby building officials inspect commercial buildings when they are first built. This system can be extended to include periodic inspections of such buildings with attention given to ventilation rates in occupied spaces rather than in supply ducts only.

Consumer Product Safety Commission

There are several federal agencies that could have the power to influence directly the quality of the indoor air we breathe, including the EPA, the Consumer Product Safety Commission (CPSC), and the Occupational Safety and Health Administration (OSHA). The EPA supports research on the indoor air environment but has not promulgated any rules concerning indoor air. The CPSC, on the other hand, already plays a significant role in regulating consumer products that have the ability to pollute the indoor air environment. OSHA may establish new air quality standards for office environments. The Department of Energy and the Department of Housing and Urban Development can influence indoor air quality in buildings through weatherization program requirements and mobile home regulations, respectively.

The CPSC has the authority to regulate consumer products to ensure the safety of users of such products. Consumer-product safety standards may be promulgated where a standard is reasonably necessary to prevent or reduce an unreasonable risk of injury associated with the use of a product. A consumer product is defined as any article or component of an article sold for the personal use, consumption, or enjoyment of a consumer. Certain products (for example, tobacco, autos, food, and drugs) are specifically excluded from CPSC considerations because they are covered by other government agencies.

The CPSC banned the use of UF foam insulation in residential and school buildings (although the ban was overturned by a federal Court of Appeals). The commission has taken action to reduce exposure to asbestos by banning it from such consumer products as patching compounds, artificial fireplace logs, and general-use clothing. It is currently considering what action, if any, to take on kerosene heaters and particle board used in residential buildings.

The CPSC could play a larger role in regulating consumer products that emit pollutants into the indoor air. For example, it could decide that all new gas stoves should have exhaust fans that automatically turn on when the oven or burners are in use. It could also regulate allowable formaldehyde emissions from plywood and particle-board products. The commission must consider the benefits and costs of any regulation it proposes, including the public's need for the product in question. The costs of product modification and product testing, it should be remembered, are much easier to compute than the benefits of reduced pollutant emissions.

An important power of the CPSC is the authority to order manufacturers to notify the public of the hazards of using particular products. The commission can even order manufacturers to repair or replace a hazardous product. One limitation of the CPSC's powers is its restriction to consumer goods. Therefore, it is unable to rule on houses as a whole, since they are not considered to be consumer products under the Consumer Product Safety Act.

Conclusion

A twofold approach to maintaining healthful air in residential buildings requires two types of actions: consumer education and consumer-product regulation. The first step calls for preparation of literature on common indoor air quality issues. Pamphlets must be written for the average non-technically oriented person. All utility companies conducting weatherization programs should provide such information to their customers. Proper education of consumers would also allow them to choose air cleaners where appropriate to control indoor air pollutants. As discussed earlier, it appears that indoor air quality regulations are not feasible in residential buildings; source control is probably the most effective method for reducing exposure to pollutants.

Since indoor air pollutant concentrations are highly dependent on the strength of pollutant sources in buildings, the CPSC can play a significant role in reducing human exposure to harmful air pollutants. Regulation of combustion appliances, such as gas stoves and kerosene heaters, is within the scope of the commission's authority. Combustion products emitted by cigarettes are not controllable by the CPSC; however, in public buildings, state and city regulations are being used effectively to separate smokers and nonsmokers. Such regulations are applicable—and rightfully so —to nonresidential buildings only. Hazardous substances such as asbestos and formaldehyde can also be controlled by CPSC rulings on products emitting these pollutants.

In commercial and institutional buildings, determination of ventilation system efficiencies, if properly done on a periodic basis, will help to alleviate some cases of tight-building syndrome. Separation of smokers and nonsmokers will also improve occupant comfort significantly. Judicious choice of building materials and furnishings will reduce emissions of hazardous substances into the indoor air. Finally, serious consideration of employee complaints should help in identifying the substances or environmental conditions causing illness or discomfort in problem buildings.

Appendixes

A

Mass-Balance Model for Indoor Air Contaminants

The concentration of an indoor air contaminant can be determined as a function of time by considering the sources and sinks of that contaminant. The potential sources are the outdoor air and indoor generators (such as formaldehyde from plywood or carbon dioxide from people) of the contaminant under consideration. The sinks are removal processes such as ventilation (mechanical or natural), infiltration, and physical and chemical processes (such as adsorption of particulates on indoor surfaces). For the purpose of simplification, the contaminant removal rate by chemical and physical processes is assumed to be proportional to the indoor concentration. The differential equation resulting from the addition of the four terms described above follows:

$$\frac{dC_i}{dt} = S/V + PC_0Q - C_iQ - kC_i \qquad (1)$$

where V is the room volume (in m^3); S the contaminant source strength (in mg/h); C_i and C_0 the contaminant concentration in the inside air and the outside air, respectively (in mg/m^3); Q air change rate (in air changes per hour) for ventilation air that enters through a mechanical ventilation system or air that infiltrates through openings in the building shell; P the fraction of outdoor air that penetrates the mechanical ventilation system or the building shell; k the rate of air contaminant removal by interaction with indoor surfaces or by chemical reaction; and t the elapsed time (in hours). Assuming S is constant and in well-mixed indoor air, the solution to the above equation is

$$C_i(t) = \frac{PQC_0 + S/V}{(Q + k)} (1 - e^{-(Q + k)t} + C_i(0)e^{-(Q + k)t}) \qquad (2)$$

Providing that S remains constant, the equilibrium contaminant concentration, $C_i(\infty)$, is attained as t goes to infinity:

$$C_i(\infty) = \frac{PQC_0 + S/V}{(Q + k)}$$

We can discuss two typical situations where it is useful to be able to approximate the equilibrium contaminant concentration. The first is where the contaminant concentration is dominated by an outdoor source. In this case, $S/V <<$ PQC_0, and thus

$$C_i(\infty) \approx PC_0/(1 + k/Q)$$

If $k = 0$, $C_i(\infty) = PC_0$; and if $P = 1$, $C_i(\infty) = C_0$. For this situation the indoor concentration eventually reaches the same value as the outdoor concentration.

The second case is where the contaminant concentration is dominated by an indoor source. In this case, $S/V >> PQC_0$, and thus

$$C_i(\infty) \approx \frac{S}{V(Q + k)}$$

if S is a constant. If $k = 0$, then $C_i(\infty)$ is inversely proportional to the ventilation rate, Q. This is an often-quoted result; nevertheless, it is only true where the steady-state value of the contaminant is concerned and where the only removal process is ventilation or infiltration.

For situations where S, the contaminant generation rate, is not constant, the solution to equation (1) is not given by equation (2) and depends upon the exact form of $S(t)$.

B

Addresses of Manufacturers and Distributors

Sources of formaldehyde detectors:

Air Quality Research, 901 Grayson Street, Berkeley, CA 94710
National Indoor Environmental Institute, 5200 Butler Pike, Plymouth Meeting, PA 19462
3M Company, P.O. Box 43157, St. Paul, MN 55164

Radon measurement services:

National Indoor Environmental Institute, 5200 Butler Pike, Plymouth Meeting, PA 19462, (215) 825-6000. This institute supplies two Terradex radon detectors and performs the analysis for about $100 (in 1984).
Terradex Corporation, 460 Wiget Lane, Walnut Creek, CA 94598, (415) 938-2545. Terradex performs eight measurements (four soil gas, two indoors, and two of radon in water) for about $100 (in 1984).

U.S. and Canadian distributors of air-to-air heat exchangers:

Berner International (for Sharp Corporation), 12 Sixth Road, Woburn, MA 01801
R. W. Besant, Department of Mechanical Engineering, University of Saskatchewan, Saskatoon, Saskatchewan, Canada S7N 0W0
Fulton M. Cook, Flakt Products, Inc. (for Svenska Flaktfabriken), P.O. Box 21500, Fort Lauderdale, FL 33335
Ray Kollock, Automated Control Systems, 500 East Higgins Road, Elk Grove, IL 60007
Melco Sales, Inc. (for Mitsubishi Electric Corp.), 3030 E. Victoria Street, Compton, CA 90221
Dennis D. Rogoza, Enercon Projects, Ltd., 2073 Cornwall Street, Regina, Saskatchewan, Canada S4P 2K6

Manufacturers of air ionizers:

Air Ion Devices, P.O. Box 2609, San Rafael, CA 94912
Amcor Group, Ltd., Empire State Building, Suite 1907, New York, NY 10001

California Air Environments, 1299 Old Bayshore Highway, Suite #110–112, Burlingame, CA 94010, (415) 342-2785

DEV Industries, Inc., 5721 Arapahoe Avenue, Boulder, CO 80303

Ion Research Center, 14670 Highway Nine, P.O. Box 905, Boulder Creek, CA 95006

ISI, 940 Dwight Way, Berkeley, CA 94710, (415) 548-3640

Light Farce, dist. Marjory Hughes, 4530 South 5th Avenue, Sp. E-2, Pocatello, ID 83204

Zestron, Inc., Department P-12, 667 McGlincey Lane, Campbell, CA 95008

Manufacturers of electronic precipitators:

Aercology, Inc., Custom Park, Old Saybrook, CT 06475

Air Control Industries, Inc., 213 McLemore Street, Nashville, TN 37203

Ammerman Company, Inc., 201 South Third Street, Hopkins, MN 55343, (612) 933-7474

Biotech Electronics, P.O. Box 14, Paterson, NJ 07507

Five Seasons Comfort Limited, 400 Eddystone Avenue, Downsview, Ontario, Canada M3N 1H7, (416) 742-0601

Honeywell, Inc., 10400 Yellow Circle Drive, Minnetonka, MN 55343

Oreck Corp., 100 Plantation Road, New Orleans, LA 70123, (504) 733-8761

Santek, Inc., P.O. Box 7934, 4110 Romaine Street, Greensboro, NC 17407, (919) 292-6909

Smokemaster, Inc., 965 North County Road 18, Minneapolis, MN 55441

Trion, Inc., P.O. Box 760, Sanford, NC 27330, (919) 775-2201

C

Addresses of Relevant Federal and State Offices

Regional Offices of the Occupational Safety and Health Administration (OSHA):

Region 1. *Boston Regional Office* (Connecticut, Maine, Massachusetts, New Hampshire, Rhode Island, and Vermont)
   Donald MacKenzie, Regional Administrator, U.S. Department of Labor–OSHA, 16–18 North Street, 1 Dock Square Building, 4th Floor, Boston, MA 02109, (617) 223-6710

Region 2. *New York Regional Office* (New Jersey, New York, and Puerto Rico)
   Byron Chadwick, Acting Regional Administrator, U.S. Department of Labor–OSHA, 1515 Broadway (1 Astor Plaza), Room 3445, New York, NY 10036, (212) 944-3426

Region 3. *Philadelphia Regional Office* (Delaware, District of Columbia, Maryland, Pennsylvania, Virginia, and West Virginia)
   David H. Rhone, Regional Administrator, U.S. Department of Labor–OSHA, Gateway Building, Suite 2100, 3535 Market Street, Philadelphia, PA 19104, (215) 596-1201

Region 4. *Atlanta Regional Office* (Alabama, Florida, Georgia, Kentucky, Mississippi, North Carolina, South Carolina, and Tennessee)
   William W. Gordon, Regional Administrator, U.S. Department of Labor–OSHA, 1375 Peachtree Street, NE, Suite 587, Atlanta, GA 30367, (404) 881-3573

Region 5. *Chicago Regional Office* (Indiana, Illinois, Michigan, Minnesota, Ohio, and Wisconsin)
   Alan C. McMillan, Regional Administrator, U.S. Department of Labor–OSHA, 32nd Floor, Room 3244, 230 South Dearborn Street, Chicago, IL 60604, (312) 353-2220

Region 6. *Dallas Regional Office* (Arkansas, Louisiana, New Mexico, Oklahoma, and Texas)
   Gilbert J. Saulter, Regional Administrator, U.S. Department of Labor–OSHA, 555 Griffin Square Building, Room 602, Dallas, TX 75202, (214) 767-4731

Region 7. *Kansas City Regional Office* (Iowa, Kansas, Missouri, and Nebraska)
Roger A. Clark, Regional Administrator, U.S. Department of Labor–OSHA, 911 Walnut Street, Room 406, Kansas City, MO 64106, (816) 374-5861

Region 8. *Denver Regional Office* (Colorado, Montana, North Dakota, South Dakota, Utah, and Wyoming)
James Lake, Acting Regional Administrator, U.S. Department of Labor–OSHA, Federal Building, Room 1554, 1961 Stout Street, Denver, CO 80294, (303) 837-3883

Region 9. *San Francisco Regional Office* (American Samoa, Arizona, California, Guam, Hawaii, Nevada, and Trust Territory of the Pacific Islands)
Gabriel Gillotti, Regional Administrator, U.S. Department of Labor–OSHA, 11349 Federal Building, 450 Golden Gate Avenue, P.O. Box 36017, San Francisco, CA 94102, (415) 556-0586

Region 10. *Seattle Regional Office* (Alaska, Idaho, Oregon, and Washington)
Frank Strasheim, Acting Regional Administrator, U.S. Department of Labor–OSHA, Federal Office Building, Room 6003, 909 1st Avenue, Seattle, WA 98174, (206) 442-5930

Central offices of states with air-quality plans approved by OSHA:

Alaska
Edmund N. Orbeck, Commissioner, Alaska Department of Labor, P.O. Box 1149, Juneau, AK 99811, (907) 465-2700

Arizona
Larry Etchechury, Director, Division of Occupational Safety and Health, Industrial Commission of Arizona, P.O. Box 19070, Phoenix, AZ 85005, (602) 255-5795

California
Donald Vial, Director, California Department of Industrial Relations, 525 Golden Gate Avenue, San Francisco, CA 94102, (415) 557-3356

Connecticut
P. Joseph Peraro, Commissioner, Connecticut Department of Labor, 200 Folly Brook Boulevard, Wethersfield, CT 06109, (203) 566-5123

Hawaii
Joshua C. Agsalud, Director, Hawaii Department of Labor and Industrial Relations, 825 Mililani Street, Honolulu, HI 96813, (808) 548-3150

Indiana
Howard E. Williams, Commissioner, Indiana Division of Labor, 1013 State Office Building, 100 North Senate Avenue, Indianapolis, IN 46204, (317) 232-2663

Iowa
Allen J. Meier, Commissioner, Iowa Bureau of Labor, State House, 307 East Seventh Street, Des Moines, IA 50319, (515) 281-3447

Kentucky
John Calhoun Wells, Commissioner, Kentucky Department of Labor, U.S. Highway 127 South, Frankfort, KY 40601, (502) 564-3070

Maryland
Harvey A. Epstein, Commissioner, Maryland Division of Labor and Industry,

Department of Licensing and Regulation, 203 E. Baltimore Street, Baltimore, MD 21202, (301) 659-4176

Michigan
William Long, Director, Michigan Department of Labor, 7150 Harris Drive, Box 30015, Lansing, MI 48909, (517) 373-9600

Dr. Bailus Walker, Director, Michigan Department of Public Health, 3500 North Logan Street, Box 30035, Lansing, MI 48909, (517) 373-1320

Minnesota
Russell B. Swanson, Commissioner, Minnesota Department of Labor and Industry, 444 Lafayette Road, St. Paul, MN 55101, (612) 296-2342

Nevada
Alan Traenkner, Director, Nevada Department of Occupational Safety and Health, Nevada Industrial Commission, 515 East Musser Street, Carson City, NV 89714, (702) 885-5240

New Mexico
Thomas E. Baca, Director, New Mexico Occupational Health and Safety Bureau, Health and Environment Department, 1480 St. Francis Drive, Santa Fe, NM 87504-0968, (505) 827-5273

North Carolina
John C. Brooks, Commissioner, North Carolina Department of Labor, P.O. Box 27407, 4 West Edenton Street, Raleigh, NC 27601, (919) 733-7166

Oregon
Roy G. Green, Director, Workers' Compensation Department, Labor and Industries Building, Salem, OR 97310, (503) 378-3304

Puerto Rico
Pedro Barez Rosario, Secretary of Labor and Human Resources, Puerto Rico Department of Labor, Prudencio Rivera Martinez Building, 505 Munoz Rivera Avenue, Hato Rey, PR 00918, (807) 754-2119/22

South Carolina
Edgar L. McGowan, Commissioner, South Carolina Department of Labor, 3600 Forest Drive, P.O. Box 11329, Columbia, SC 29211, (803) 758-2851

Tennessee
J. B. Richesin, Jr., Commissioner, Tennessee Department of Labor, Attn: Robert Taylor, 501 Union Bldg, Suite "A," 2nd Floor, Nashville, TN 37219, (612) 741-2582

Utah
Walter T. Axelgard, Commissioner, Utah Industrial Commission, 350 East 5th South, Salt Lake City, UT 84111, (801) 533-4415

Vermont
Dean B. Pineles, Commissioner, Vermont Department of Labor and Industry, 118 State Street, Montpelier, VT 05602, (802) 828-2765

Virginia
Robert F. Beard, Jr., Commissioner, Virginia Department of Labor and Industry, P.O. Box 12064, Richmond, VA 23241, (804) 786-2376

Dr. James B. Kenley, Commissioner, Virginia Department of Health, James Madison Building, 109 Governor Street, Richmond, VA 23219, (804) 936-4265

Virgin Islands
> Richard Upson, Commissioner of Labor, Government of Virgin Islands, Box 890, Christiansted, St. Croix, VI 00820, (809) 773-1994

Washington
> Samuel Kinville, Director, Washington Department of Labor and Industries, General Administration Building, Room 334—AX-31, Olympia, WA 98504, (206) 753-6307

Wyoming
> Donald Owsley, Administrator, Department of Occupational Safety and Health, 200 East Eighth Avenue, Cheyenne, WY 82002, (307) 777-7786

Sources and
Suggested Reading

Sources and Suggested Reading

1 Introduction

Notes

1. C. H. Hales, S. M. Rollinson, and F. H. Shair, "Experimental Verification of Linear Combination Model for Relating Indoor-Outdoor Pollutant Concentrations," *Environmental Science and Technology*, vol. 8, no. 5 (May 1974).

2. J. V. Berk *et al.*, *Indoor Air Quality Measurements in Energy-Efficient Residential Buildings*, Lawrence Berkeley Laboratory Report LBL-8894 (1980).

Suggestions for Further Reading

All About OSHA. Washington, DC: U.S. Department of Labor, Occupational Safety and Health Administration, 1982. Available from OSHA Publications Distribution, Room S-1212, Washington, DC 20210.

"E.P.A. Sets National Air Quality Standards." *Air Pollution Control Association Journal* 21: 352–53 (June 1971).

Indoor Air Quality Handbook: For Designers, Builders, and Users of Energy Efficient Residences. Prepared for the Department of Energy. Albuquerque, NM: Sandia National Laboratories and AnaChem, Inc., 1982. Available from National Technical Information Service, 5285 Port Royal Road, Springfield, VA 22161.

Meyer, B. *Indoor Air Quality*. New York: Addison-Wesley, 1983.

National Research Council. *Indoor Pollutants*. Washington, DC: National Academy Press, 1981.

Proceedings of the International Symposium on Indoor Air Pollution, Health and Energy Conservation. Special issue. *Environment International*, vol. 8, nos. 1–6 (1982).

Stern, Arthur, ed. *Air Pollution; Volume 1, Air Pollution and Its Effects*. New York: Academic Press, 1968.

"Symposium on Health Aspects of Indoor Air Pollution." *Bulletin of the New York Academy of Medicine*, vol. 57, no. 10 (December 1981).

Wadden, R. A., and P. A. Schiff. *Indoor Air Pollution: Characterization, Prediction, and Control*. New York: Wiley, 1983.

2 Formaldehyde and Other Household Contaminants

Notes

1. "The Danger Within," *ABC News 20/20*, broadcast February 4, 1982.

2. National Research Council, *Formaldehyde and Other Aldehydes* (Washington, DC: National Academy Press, 1981).

3. Committee on Toxicology, National Research Council, *Formaldehyde—An Assessment of Its Health Effects* (Washington, DC: National Academy Press, 1980).

4. L. Levin and P. W. Purdom, "A Review of the Health Effects of Energy Conserving Materials," *American Journal of Public Health*, vol. 73, no. 6 (June 1983).

5. Connecticut Department of Consumer Protection, *Governor's Task Force on Insulation: Report on UF Foam Insulation* (Hartford: State of Connecticut, 1978).

6. *Status Report on the Indoor Air Quality Monitoring Study in 40 Homes*, Oak Ridge National Laboratory (1984).

7. Memorandum from 3M Company, Occupational Health and Safety Products Division, St. Paul, MN (1982).

8. J. C. Harris *et al.*, "Toxicology of Urea-Formaldehyde and Polyurethane Foam Insulation," *Journal of the American Medical Association*, vol. 245, no. 3 (January 1981).

9. P. A. Breysse, "The Environmental Problems of UF Structures—Formaldehyde Exposure in Mobile Homes," presented at the Occupational Safety and Health Symposium of the American Medical Association, June 1980.

10. See note 1.

11. J. F. van der Wal, "Formaldehyde Measurements in Dutch Houses, Schools, and Offices," *Atmospheric Environment* 16: 2471–78 (1982).

12. "A Flood of Lawsuits over Formaldehyde Insulation," *San Francisco Chronicle*, June 9, 1982.

13. *Urea-Formaldehyde Foam Insulation*, U.S. Consumer Product Safety Commission (1982).

14. R. A. Jewell, *Reduction of Formaldehyde Levels in Mobile Homes* (Tacoma, WA: Weyerhaeuser Company, 1980).

Suggestions for Further Reading

"Urea-Formaldehyde Foam Insulation" and other literature on formaldehyde can be obtained from several sources: U.S. Consumer Product Safety Commission at 1111 Eighteenth Street NW, Washington, DC 20207, or 5401 Westbard Avenue, Bethesda, MD 20207, hotline: (800) 638-8326; Formaldehyde Institute, 1075 Central Park Avenue, Scarsdale, NY 10583, (914) 725-1492; and S.U.F.F.E.R. (Save Us From Formaldehyde Environmental Repercussions), c/o Connie Smrecek, National S.U.F.F.E.R. Coordinator, RR Box 148C, Waconia, MN 55387, (612) 448-5441. When requesting information from S.U.F.F.E.R., send a self-addressed stamped envelope.

California Department of Consumer Affairs. *Clean Your Room*, Chapter 3C. Sacramento, CA: State of California, 1982.

National Research Council. *Indoor Pollutants*, Chapters 4 and 7. Washington, DC: National Academy Press, 1981.

3 Radon

Notes

1. "Warning: Home Energy Conservation May Be Dangerous to Your Health," *National Journal*, no. 31 (August 2, 1980).

2. B. Peterson, *Field Surveys of Phosphate Slag Used for Construction Purposes in Idaho Springs, Idaho* (Boise: Idaho Department of Health and Welfare, 1979).

3. O. Hildingson, *Measurements of Radon Daughters in 5600 Swedish Homes* (Boras: Swedish National Testing Institute, Division of Building Physics, 1981).

4. H. W. Alter, *Indoor Radon Levels: Field Experience Using the Track Etch ®️ Method* (Walnut Creek, CA: Terradex Corporation, 1981).

5. A. V. Nero, Jr., *Indoor Radiation Exposures from Radon and Its Daughters: A View of the Issues*, Lawrence Berkeley Laboratory Report LBL-10525 (1981).

6. A. V. Nero et al., *Radon Concentrations and Infiltration Rates Measured in Conventional and Energy-Efficient Houses*, Lawrence Berkeley Laboratory Report LBL-13415 (1981).

7. *Study of Radon Daughter Concentrations in Structures in Polk and Hillsborough Counties*, Florida Department of Health and Rehabilitative Services, Radiological Health Services (1978).

8. National Research Council, *Indoor Pollutants* (Washington, DC: National Academy Press, 1981), Chapter 7.

9. *Ibid.*, Chapter 7, Table 7-2.

10. E. Stranden, "Radon in Dwellings and Lung Cancer—A Discussion," *Health Physics* 38: 301–6 (March 1980).

11. W. W. Nazaroff et al., "The Use of Mechanical Ventilation with Heat Recovery for Controlling Radon and Radon-Daughter Concentrations in Houses," *Atmospheric Environment* 15: 263–70 (1981).

Suggestions for Further Reading

Health Physics, vol. 45, no. 2 (August 1983). Special issue on indoor radon.

National Research Council. *Indoor Pollutants*, Chapters 4 and 7. Washington, DC: National Academy Press, 1981.

Nero, A. V., Jr. *Indoor Radiation Exposures from Radon and Its Daughters: A View of the Issues.* Lawrence Berkeley Laboratory Report LBL-10525 (1981).

Proceedings of the International Symposium on Indoor Air Pollution, Health and Energy Conservation, Sessions B1 and D1. Special issue. *Environment International*, vol. 8, nos. 1–6 (1982).

4 Particulates

Notes

1. A. P. Krueger and E. J. Reed, "Biological Impact of Small Air Ions," *Science* 193: 1209–13 (September 24, 1976).

2. F. Sulman, "Air Ionometry of Hot, Dry Desert Winds (Sharav) and Treatment with Air Ions of Weather-Sensitive Subjects," *International Journal of Biometeorology* 4: 101–10 (1963).

3. Literature provided by California Air Environments, 1299 Bayshore Highway, Burlingame, CA 94010.

4. *Ibid.*

5. T. A. David, J. R. Minehart, and I. H. Kornblueh, "Polarized Air as an Adjunct in the Treatment of Burns," *American Journal of Physical Medicine* 39: 111–13 (1960).

6. "Asbestos Danger at Federal Building," *San Francisco Examiner*, January 9, 1983.

7. I. J. Selikoff, "Household Risks with Inorganic Fibers," Symposium on Health Aspects of Indoor Air Pollution, *Bulletin of the New York Academy of Medicine*, vol. 57, no. 10 (December 1981).

8. "Home Furnace Asbestos—State's Hidden Danger," *San Francisco Chronicle*, January 18, 1983.

9. "Fiberglass Cleared of Health Hazards," *Energy Conservation Digest*, vol. 6, no. 2 (January 17, 1983).

10. M. A. Chatigny and R. L. Dimmick, "Transport of Aerosols in the Intramural Environment," in R. L. Edmonds, ed., *Aerobiology: The Ecological System Approach* (Stroudsburg, PA: Dowden, Hutchinson & Ross, 1979).

11. R. C. Riley *et al.*, "Airborne Spread of Measles in a Suburban Elementary School," *American Journal of Epidemiology* 107: 421–32 (1978).

12. D. W. Alling *et al.*, "A Study of Excess Mortality During Influenza Epidemics in the United States, 1968–1976," *American Journal of Epidemiology* 113: 30–43 (1981).

13. G. H. Green, "The Positive and Negative Effects of Building Humidification," *ASHRAE Transactions*, vol. 88 (1982).

14. G. Ewert, "On the Mucus Flow Rate in the Human Nose," *Acta Oto Laryng Stockholm* 21: 56 (1965).

15. I. Andersen, in *Proceedings of the 1978 International Working Conference on Hospital Ventilation Standards and Energy Conservation*, Lawrence Berkeley Laboratory Report LBL-8257 (1978).

Suggestions for Further Reading

Edmonds, R. L., ed. *Aerobiology: The Ecological System Approach.* Stroudsburg, PA: Dowden, Hutchinson & Ross, 1979.

National Research Council. *Indoor Pollutants*, Chapters 4 and 7. Washington, DC: National Academy Press, 1981.

Soyka, F., with A. Edmonds. *The Ion Effect.* New York: Bantam Books, 1977.

5   Combustion Products

Notes

1. R. A. Ziskind *et al.*, "Carbon Monoxide Intrusion into Sustained-Use Vehicles," *Environment International* 5: 109–23 (1981).

2. National Research Council, *Indoor Pollutants* (Washington, DC: National Academy Press, 1981).

3. *Ibid.*

4. T. D. Sterling and D. Kobayashi, "Use of Gas Ranges for Cooking and Heating in Urban Dwellings," *Air Pollution Control Association Journal*, vol. 31, no. 2 (February 1981).

5. G. W. Traynor *et al.*, *The Effects of Ventilation on Residential Air Pollution*

Due to Emissions from a Gas-Fired Range, Lawrence Berkeley Laboratory Report LBL-12563 (1981).

6. T. D. Sterling and E. Sterling, "Carbon Monoxide Levels in Kitchens and Homes with Gas Cookers," *Air Pollution Control Association Journal*, vol. 29, no. 3 (March 1979).

7. See note 5.

8. "Pollution Danger in India's Homes," *Honolulu Star Bulletin*, November 12, 1982.

9. A. L. Aggarwal *et al.*, "Assessment of Exposure to Benzo-*a*-pyrene in Air for Various Population Groups in Ahmedabad," *Atmospheric Environment* 16: 867–70 (1982).

10. T. D. Sterling, J. Weinkam, and E. Sterling, "The Case for Entirely Removing the Gas Range from Indoors," *Proceedings of the International Symposium on Indoor Air Pollution, Health and Energy Conservation*, Session G, special issue of *Environment International*, vol. 8, nos. 1–6 (1982).

11. R. J. Melia, C. du V. Florey, and S. Chinn, "The Relationship Between Respiratory Illness in Primary Schoolchildren and the Use of Gas for Cooking," *International Journal of Epidemiology* 8(4): 333–53 (1979).

12. F. E. Speizer *et al.*, "Respiratory Disease Rates and Pulmonary Function in Children Associated with Nitrogen Dioxide Exposure," *American Review of Respiratory Disease* 121: 3–10 (1980).

13. V. Hasselblad *et al.*, "Indoor Environmental Determinants of Lung Function in Children," *American Review of Respiratory Disease* 123: 479–85 (1981).

14. K. J. Helsing *et al.*, "Respiratory Effects of Household Exposures to Tobacco Smoke and Gas Cooking on Non-Smokers," *Proceedings of the International Symposium on Indoor Air Pollution, Health and Energy Conservation*, Session D1, special issue of *Environment International*, vol. 8, nos. 1–6 (1982).

15. M. D. Keller *et al.*, "Respiratory Illness in Households Using Gas and Electricity for Cooking," *Environmental Research* 19: 495–515 (1979).

16. *Ibid.*

17. See note 5.

18. "Are Kerosene Heaters Safe?" *Consumer Reports*, October 1982.

19. J. G. Girman *et al.*, *Pollutant Emission Rates from Indoor Combustion Appliances and Sidestream Cigarette Smoke*, Lawrence Berkeley Laboratory Report LBL-12562 (1981).

20. B. P. Leaderer, "Air Pollutant Emissions from Kerosene Space Heaters," *Science*, vol. 218 (December 10, 1982).

21. "Popular Kerosene Heaters Stir U.S. Concern on Safety," *New York Times*, October 28, 1982.

22. See note 19.

23. D. J. Moschandreas, J. Zabransky, and H. E. Rector, "The Effects of Woodburning on the Indoor Residential Air Quality," *Environment International* 4: 463–68 (1980).

24. *Ibid.*

Suggestions for Further Reading

"Are Kerosene Heaters Safe?" *Consumer Reports*, October 1982.

Fox, J., C. Hall, and L. Elveback. *Epidemiology, Man and Disease*. New York: Macmillan, 1972.

"Hotter Competition for the Heater Leader." *Fortune*, March 8, 1982.

National Research Council. *Indoor Pollutants*, Chapters 4 and 7. Washington, DC: National Academy Press, 1981.

Proceedings of the International Symposium on Indoor Air Pollution, Health and Energy Conservation, Sessions C2 and D1. Special issue. *Environment International*, vol. 8, nos. 1–6 (1982).

Twitchell, M. *Wood Energy, a Practical Guide to Heating with Wood.* Charlotte, VT: Garden Way, 1978.

6 Involuntary Smoking

Notes

1. *Shimp v. Bell Telephone Company*, 145 N.J. Super. 516, 568 A2d 48 (App. Div. 1976).

2. "Burned up Bosses Snuff Out Prospects of Jobs for Smokers," *Wall Street Journal*, April 15, 1982.

3. W. L. Weiss and C. P. Fleenor, "Cold-Shouldering the Smoker," *Supervisory Management*, September 1981.

4. National Research Council, *Indoor Pollutants* (Washington, DC: National Academy Press, 1981), Chapter 4.

5. R. T. Ravenholt, "Letter to the Editor," *New England Journal of Medicine*, July 29, 1982.

6. J. L. Repace and A. H. Lowrey, "Indoor Air Pollution, Tobacco Smoke, and Public Health," *Science*, vol. 208 (May 2, 1980).

7. J. D. Spengler *et al.*, "Long-Term Measurements of Respirable Sulfates and Particles Inside and Outside Homes," *Atmospheric Environment* 15: 23–30 (1981).

8. "Study Finds New Threat to Smokers," *San Francisco Chronicle*, March 18, 1982.

9. Examples include these two: S. Harlap and A. M. Davis, "Infant Admissions to Hospitals and Maternal Smoking," *The Lancet* 1: 529–32 (1974); and J. R. Colley *et al.*, "Influence of Passive Smoking and Parental Phlegm on Pneumonia and Bronchitis in Early Childhood," *The Lancet* 2: 1031–34 (1974).

10. G. S. Bonham and R. W. Wilson, "Children's Health in Families with Cigarette Smokers," *American Journal of Public Health*, vol. 171, no. 3 (March 1981).

11. I. B. Tager *et al.*, "The Effect of Parental Cigarette Smoking on the Pulmonary Function of Children," *American Journal of Epidemiology* 110(1): 15–29 (1979).

12. J. R. White and H. F. Froeb, "Small-Airways Dysfunction in Nonsmokers Chronically Exposed to Tobacco Smoke," *New England Journal of Medicine* 302: 720–23 (1980).

13. F. Kauffmann, "Small Airways Dysfunction in Nonsmokers," *New England Journal of Medicine* 303: 393–400 (1980).

14. C. B. Barad, "Smoking on the Job: The Controversy Heats Up," *Occupational Health and Safety* 48: 21–24 (1979).

15. "Smoking and Cancer in the United States," *Preventive Medicine* 9: 169–73 (1980).

16. *The Health Consequences of Smoking*, report of the Surgeon General (Washington, DC: U.S. Department of Health and Human Services, Public Health Services, 1981).

17. E. C. Hammond, *Smoking in Relation to the Death Rates of 100,000 Men and Women*, National Cancer Institute Monograph 19 (1966).

18. T. Hirayama, "Nonsmoking Wives of Heavy Smokers Have a Higher Risk of Lung Cancer: A Study from Japan," *British Medical Journal* 282: 183–85 (January 17, 1981).

19. G. H. Miller, "Letter to the Editor," *British Medical Journal* 282: 1156 (March 21, 1981).

20. T. D. Sterling, "Letter to the Editor," *British Medical Journal* 282: 1156 (March 21, 1981).

21. *Ibid.*

22. E. Grundmann, K. M. Müller, and K. D. Winter, "Letter to the Editor," *British Medical Journal* 282: 1157 (March 21, 1981).

23. D. Trichopoulos *et al.*, "Lung Cancer and Passive Smoking," *International Journal of Cancer*, vol. 27 (1981).

24. P. Correa *et al.*, "Passive Smoking and Lung Cancer," *The Lancet*, September 10, 1983, pp. 595–97.

25. *Before You Believe Half the Story, Get the Whole Story; Case in Point: The Public Smoking Issue*, The Tobacco Institute, August 1981.

26. L. Garfinkel, "Time Trends in Lung Cancer Mortality Among Nonsmokers: A Note on Passive Smoking," *Journal of the National Cancer Institute* 66(6): 1061–66 (June 1981).

Suggestions for Further Reading

The Health Consequences of Smoking. Report of the Surgeon General. Washington, DC: U.S. Department of Health and Human Services, Public Health Services, 1981.

National Research Council. *Indoor Pollutants*, Chapters 4 and 7. Washington, DC: National Academy Press, 1981.

Shimp, D., *et al. How to Protect Your Health at Work*. Salem, NJ: Environmental Improvement Associates, 1976.

7 Energy-Efficient Buildings and Indoor Air Quality

Notes

1. D. T. Grimsrud, R. D. Lipschutz, and J. R. Girman, "Energy Efficient Residences," in C. Dudley, ed., *Indoor Air Quality* (Chemical Rubber Company, 1984).

2. A. V. Nero *et al.*, *Radon Concentrations and Infiltration Rates Measured in Conventional and Energy-Efficient Houses*, Lawrence Berkeley Laboratory Report LBL-13415 (1981).

3. *National Energy Conservation Policy Act*, PL95–619.

4. "BPA Weighs All-Out Program," *Energy Conservation Digest*, December 20, 1982.

5. A. V. Nero, I. Turiel, W. Fisk, J. Girman, and G. W. Traynor, *Exclusion List Methodology for Weatherization Program in the Pacific Northwest*, Lawrence Berkeley Laboratory Report LBL-14467 (1982).

6. *The House Doctor's Manual*, Lawrence Berkeley Laboratory Publication 3017, and *Find and Fix the Leaks*, Publication 384, both prepared for the Department of Energy (Washington, DC: Government Printing Office, 1981).

Suggestions for Further Reading

Find and Fix the Leaks. Prepared for the Department of Energy. Lawrence Berkeley Laboratory Publication 384 (1981).

The House Doctor's Manual. Prepared for the Department of Energy. Lawrence Berkeley Laboratory Publication 3017 (1981).

Norback, P., and C. Norback. *The Consumer's Energy Handbook.* New York: Van Nostrand, 1981.

8 Control of Indoor Air Pollutants

Notes

1. W. J. Fisk and I. Turiel, "Residential Air to Air Heat Exchangers: Performance, Energy Savings and Economics," *Energy and Buildings* 5: 197–211 (1983).

2. K. Alder, C. D. Hollowell, and W. J. Fisk, *Control of Formaldehyde and Radon in the Built Environment: A Survey of the Literature,* Lawrence Berkeley Laboratory Report LBID-625 (1982).

3. "A Test of Small Air Cleaners," *New Shelter,* July–August 1982.

4. F. J. Offermann *et al., Control of Respirable Particulates and Radon Progeny with Portable Air Cleaners,* Lawrence Berkeley Laboratory Report LBL-16659 (1983).

5. W. S. Cain and B. P. Leaderer, "Ventilation Requirements in Occupied Spaces During Smoking and Nonsmoking Occupancy," *Environment International* 8: 505–14 (1982).

Suggestions for Further Reading

Alder, K., C. D. Hollowell, and W. J. Fisk. *Control of Formaldehyde and Radon in the Built Environment: A Survey of the Literature.* Lawrence Berkeley Laboratory Report LBID-625 (1982).

Shurcliff, W. A. *Air-to-Air Heat Exchangers for Houses.* Cambridge, MA: the author, 1981. Available from the author, 19 Appleton Street, Cambridge, MA 02100.

"A Test of Small Air Cleaners," *New Shelter,* July–August 1982.

9 Indoor Air Quality Problems in Office Buildings

Notes

1. S. Blakeslee, "Buildings That Make You Sick," *San Francisco Chronicle,* June 15, 1980.

2. R. Johnson, "Mystery Plague Forces NBC Workers to Quit Jobs," *New York Post,* September 30, 1981.

3. R. A. Keenlyside, *Recent NIOSH Investigations of Complaints of Uncertain Etiology Affecting Workers in Closed Office Areas,* National Institute of Occupational Safety and Health, Hazard Evaluations and Technical Assistance Branch, Cincinnati, OH (1980).

4. *Standards for Natural and Mechanical Ventilation,* American Society of Heating, Refrigeration, and Air-Conditioning Engineers (ASHRAE) Publication 62-73R (1973).

5. C. P. Yaglou *et al.,* "Ventilation Requirements," *Transactions of the American Society of Heating and Ventilating Engineers* 42: 132–62 (1936).

6. I. Turiel *et al.,* "The Effects of Reduced Ventilation on Indoor Air Quality in an Office Building," *Atmospheric Environment* 17: 51–64 (1983).

7. M. Ganier *et al.,* "Humidifier Lung, an Outbreak in Office Workers," *Chest* 77(2): 183–87 (February 1980).

8. D. W. Fraser *et al.*, "Legionnaire's Disease, Description of an Epidemic of Pneumonia," *New England Journal of Medicine*, vol. 297, no. 22 (December 1977).

9. P. J. Imperato, "Legionellosis and the Indoor Environment," *Bulletin of the New York Academy of Medicine*, vol. 57, no. 10 (December 1981).

10. K. Kreiss and M. J. Hodgson, "Building Associated Epidemics," Center for Environmental Health, Centers for Disease Control, Atlanta, GA (1982).

11. *Ibid.*

12. P. A. Patriarca *et al.*, "Kawasaki Syndrome: Association with the Application of Rug Shampoo," *The Lancet*, September 1982, pp. 578–80.

13. V. Beral *et al.*, "Malignant Melanoma and Exposure to Fluorescent Lighting at Work," *The Lancet*, August 7, 1982, pp. 290–93.

14. *In the Chips: Opportunities, People, Partnerships*, Labour Canada Task Force on Micro-Electronics and Employment, Ottawa, 1982.

15. *Potential Health Hazards of Video Display Terminals*, National Institute of Occupational Safety and Health, Cincinnati, OH (1981). See also note 14.

16. *Epidemic Respiratory Tract Irritation—Florida*, memorandum to the Director of the Centers for Disease Control from the Chronic Disease Division of the Bureau of Epidemiology, December 8, 1978.

17. S. M. Stahl and M. Lebedun, "Mystery Gas: An Analysis of Mass Hysteria," *Journal of Health and Social Behavior* 15: 44–50 (1974).

18. M. J. Colligan, "The Psychological Effects of Indoor Air Pollution," *Bulletin of the New York Academy of Medicine*, vol. 57, no. 10 (December 1981).

19. I. Turiel and J. Rudy, "Occupant-Generated Carbon Dioxide as an Indicator of Ventilation Rate," Lawrence Berkeley Laboratory Report LBL-10496 (1980).

20. Memorandum from CAL/OSHA Consultation Service Report, Sacramento, CA, May 13, 1982.

21. Conversation with Dr. Robert Miksch, University of California, Berkeley, School of Public Health.

22. J. Foote, "Court Agrees: Co-Workers' Smoke Poison to Her," *San Francisco Examiner*, October 22, 1982.

Suggestions for Further Reading

Colligan, M. J., *et al. Mass Psychogenic Illness: A Social Psychological Analysis.* Hillsdale, NJ: L. Erlbaum Associates, 1982.

Makower, John. *Office Hazards.* Washington, DC: Tilden Press, 1981.

Ott, John. *Health and Light.* New York: Pocket Books, 1973.

Stellman, J. M., and S. M. Daum. *Work Is Dangerous to Your Health.* New York: Vantage Books, 1973.

10 Legal and Regulatory Issues

Notes

1. M. Kurzman and J. Golden, "Formaldehyde Litigation: A Beginning," *Trial*, January 1983, pp. 82–85.

2. J. D. Blackburn, "Legal Aspects of Smoking in the Workplace," *Labor Law Journal*, 1980, pp. 564–69.

3. *Heritage* v. *Pioneer Homes*, Product Liability Reports, para. 8521 (1979).

4. See *Blagg* v. *Fred Hunt Co., Inc.*, 612 SW2d 321, 322 (1981).

5. See note 1.

6. M. Kurzman, A. Shapiro, J. H. Manahan, and W. S. Partridge, "Cases Concluded," Minneapolis, MN, October 1983.

7. *Wall Street Journal*, September 7, 1983, p. 33.

8. *San Francisco Chronicle*, April 25, 1982, p. 11.

9. *San Francisco Chronicle*, June 9, 1982, p. F-3.

10. See note 1.

11. M. Swingle, "Legal Conflict Between Smokers and Nonsmokers: The Majestic Vice Versus the Right to Clean Air," *Missouri Law Review*, vol. 45, p. 444 (1980).

12. *Shimp* v. *Bell Telephone Company*, 145 N.J.Super. 516, 568 A2d 48 (App. Div. 1976).

13. J. Foote, "Court Agrees: Co-Workers' Smoke Poison to Her," *San Francisco Examiner*, October 22, 1982.

Suggestions for Further Reading

Ashford, N., C. Ryan, and C. Caldart. "A Hard Look at Federal Regulation of Formaldehyde: A Departure from Reasoned Decisionmaking." *Harvard Environmental Law Review* 7: 297–370 (1983).

Indoor Air Quality Handbook: For Designers, Builders, and Users of Energy Efficient Residences, Chapter 8. Prepared for the Department of Energy. Albuquerque, NM: Sandia National Laboratories and AnaChem, Inc., 1982.

Kirsch, L. S. "Behind Closed Doors: Indoor Air Pollution and Government Policy." *Harvard Environmental Law Review* 6: 339–95 (1982).

Kurzman, M., and J. Golden. "Formaldehyde Litigation: A Beginning." *Trial*, January 1983.

Sexton, K., and R. Repetto. "Indoor Air Pollution and Public Policy." *Environment International* 8(1–6): 5–10 (1982).

Glossary

Glossary

ach   Abbreviation for air changes per hour, a unit of air exchange rate.

activated charcoal   A carbon-containing material that is prepared by destructive distillation to make it more adsorptive.

adsorption   The removal of gases or liquids from the air by their retention on the surface of a solid material.

aerosols   Solid or liquid particles that are small enough (0.01 to 100 micrometers) to remain suspended in the air for a period of time.

air cleaner   A device designed to remove atmospheric airborne impurities such as dust, smoke, and odorants.

air exchange   Movement of air into and out of a building by infiltration, exfiltration, natural ventilation, and mechanical ventilation.

air exchange rate   Amount of air that flows into or out of a building in a specified amount of time.

air filter   An air-cleaning device that removes particulate matter from the air.

aldehydes   A series of organic compounds, such as formaldehyde, characterized by the group CHO and having strong odors.

aliphatic hydrocarbon   An open-chain hydrocarbon, such as methane, propane, and butane.

alkyl group   A group of atoms that results when an aliphatic hydrocarbon loses one hydrogen atom.

alkylated aromatic hydrocarbon   A hydrocarbon of benzene-ring molecular structure in which an alkyl group has been substituted or added.

allergic   Highly susceptible to a substance that does not affect most people.

alpha particle   A positively charged particle (a helium nucleus) emitted in radioactive decay, as from radon.

alveoli   Tiny air sacs in the lungs where the process of respiration takes place: the blood takes in oxygen and gives up carbon dioxide.

ambient air   That portion of the air, external to buildings, to which the general public has access.

antibody   Substances in the body that combine with antigens to neutralize toxins, and that precipitate soluble antigens.

antigen   A substance such as pollen that stimulates the production of antibodies when it enters the body.

aromatic hydrocarbons   Organic chemicals characterized by the presence of the benzene-ring molecular structure.

asbestos   A hydrated magnesium silicate mineral (a compound containing water, magnesium, silicon, and oxygen) in fibrous form, used for fireproof insulation.

ASHRAE   American Society of Heating, Refrigeration, and Air Conditioning Engineers.

benzene   A colorless, volatile liquid hydrocarbon used as a solvent. It is toxic and acts on blood-forming organs, producing anemia and reducing the ability of the blood to clot.

breach of contract   Failure to fulfill a formal agreement.

breach of warranty   Failure of a product or process to fulfill express or implied representations or promises.

bronchial tubes   Branches or subdivisions of the trachea (windpipe).

BTU   British thermal unit, the amount of heat energy needed to raise the temperature of 1 pound of water by 1°F.

carbon dioxide   A colorless, odorless gas (CO_2) that is a product of the combustion of carbon-containing fuels and of human metabolism.

carbon monoxide   A colorless, odorless gas (CO) that is a product of incomplete combustion.

carcinogenic   Producing cancer.

cfm   Cubic feet per minute.

chlordane   A chlorinated hydrocarbon ($C_{10}H_6Cl_8$), toxic to insects and man.

chronic   Persistent, prolonged, or repeated.

combustion   Burning of a fuel such as wood or oil.

concentration   Amount of a substance in a given volume of air.

conduction   Movement of heat through a solid material.

contaminant   A substance not normally present in the atmosphere.

convection   Heat transfer in a fluid (gases or liquids) by movement of the fluid.

curie   A measure of the rate at which energy is released by a radioactive material. One gram of radium has a radioactivity of one curie (1 Ci), which is equal to the disintegrations of 37 billion nuclei per second.

daughter   A product atom resulting from the radioactive decay of the parent atom.

detergent   A substance that purifies or cleanses.

diffusion   Spontaneous movement of particulates and gas molecules throughout the air from areas of high concentration to low concentration.

dispersion   Movement of substances through the air by diffusion and mechanical mixing.

distillate   Material obtained by vaporizing a substance and condensing the vapor.

dose   Amount of energy or quantity of a substance absorbed in a part of the body or in an individual.

dyspnea   Shortness of breath; difficult or labored breathing.

efficiency   The effectiveness of a device in removing particulates from the air, often expressed as the percentage of particles originally in the air that are removed by the device.

electromagnetic radiation   Energy that is transmitted through space at the speed of light (for example, visible light, radio waves, x-rays).

electrostatic interaction   Mutual attraction or repulsion of materials that contain electrical charges of the opposite sign or like sign, respectively.

electrostatic precipitation   Removal of particulates from the air by attracting them to charged materials.

emission rate   Amount of contaminant released into the air by a source in a specified amount of time.

encapsulation   Covering of an object with a film or coating to prevent the release of air contaminants.

envelope   The exterior walls, windows, and roof enclosing the occupied space of a building.

EPA   Environmental Protection Agency, the federal agency responsible for setting and enforcing ambient air quality standards.

epidemiology   The study of disease as it spreads and involves large groups of people.

exfiltration   Uncontrolled movement of air out of a building through cracks and openings in the building envelope.

filtration   Removal of particulates from the air by passing the air through a filter.

fluids   Materials that flow; liquids and gases.

formaldehyde   An odorous gas (HCHO) emitted from many building materials that is an irritant to the eyes and respiratory system.

fungus   A plant that lacks chlorophyll and lives on other living organisms.

half-life   The time it takes for half of the atoms in a given quantity of radioactive material to decay.

heat exchanger   A device in which heat is transferred from one airstream to another without physical contact between them.

hemoglobin   The part of the blood that carries oxygen throughout the body.

HEPA   Abbreviation for high-efficiency particulate air filter.

hydrocarbon   Compounds containing only hydrogen and carbon, such as methane, the prime component of natural gas.

infectious agents   Bacteria, microorganisms, and viruses that can cause human disease.

infiltration   Uncontrolled movement of air into a building through cracks and openings in the building envelope.

inhalable particulates   Particles that are not filtered out by the nose and that may be deposited along the respiratory tract; the upper size limit is approximately 15 micrometers.

ion generator   A device that produces charged particles in the air.

ionize   To remove an electron from an atom by imparting energy and thus create charged particles (positive or negative ions).

mechanical ventilation   Forced movement of air by fans into and out of a building.

methyl chloride   A chlorinated hydrocarbon (CH_3Cl) that is a volatile anesthetic liquid.

microgram   A unit of mass equal to one-millionth of a gram.

micrometer   A unit of length equal to one-millionth of a meter.

molecule   Generally, the smallest particle of matter that has the same chemical properties as the larger mass.

naphthalene   A white crystalline hydrocarbon ($C_{10}H_8$) used as a solvent.

natural ventilation   Movement of air into and out of buildings through open doors and windows.

negligence   Failure to exercise proper care, resulting in an injury or damage to a person or property.

ng/m^3   Abbreviation for nanograms per cubic meter, a unit of concentration for particulate matter suspended in air. A nanogram is equal to one-billionth of a gram.

NIOSH   National Institute of Occupational Safety and Health.

nitric oxide   A colorless gas (NO) formed during combustion that is highly irritating to the skin, eyes, and respiratory tract.

nitrogen dioxide   A reddish-brown gas (NO_2) formed during combustion that is highly irritating to the lungs.

nitrogen oxides   Several compounds of nitrogen and oxygen (NO_x), including nitric oxide and nitrogen dioxide, that are formed during combustion.

organic compounds   Substances that contain carbon. Carbon dioxide (CO_2) is usually excepted.

OSHA   Occupational Safety and Health Administration.

outgassing   Emission of gases during the aging and degradation of a substance.

particulate   A small particle that remains suspended in air.

pollutant   A substance not normally found in air or water that may be harmful to living organisms.

ppm   Abbreviation for parts per million, a unit of concentration.

prefilter   An initial filter that removes large particles in an air cleaner.

radiation   Energy transfer by particles (such as alpha particles) or electromagnetic waves.

radon   A chemically inert gas that undergoes radioactive decay by emission of an alpha particle.

radon daughters   A series of radioactive elements that result from the radioactive decay of radon.

respirable particles   Particles that penetrate to the lungs when inhaled; the upper size limit is approximately 5 micrometers.

smoke   A mixture of gases and small particles generated by incomplete combustion.

source   An object or process that releases contaminants into the air.

strict liability   Responsibility for injury or damage in spite of the terms of a contract or warranty having been fulfilled.

suspended particles   Particles so small that they remain in the air for long time periods; the upper size limit is approximately 100 micrometers.

synergism   Simultaneous action of two or more substances where the total effect is greater than the sum of their individual effects.

toluene   A hydrocarbon ($CH_3C_6H_5$) that is a colorless liquid with a strong odor, used as a solvent.

toxicity   Ability of a substance to produce a harmful health effect after physical contact, ingestion, or inhalation.

trichloroethane   A solvent that tends to attack the central nervous system when inhaled; also called methyl chloroform ($C_2H_3Cl_3$).

trichloroethylene   A chlorinated hydrocarbon that is a colorless liquid ($CHCl:CCl_2$) used as an anesthetic.

vapor   Gaseous phase of a substance that is predominantly a liquid at room temperature.

ventilation   Controlled movement of air into and out of a building.

volatile   Tending to evaporate rapidly.

WL   Abbreviation for working level, a unit of radon-daughter concentration.

working level   Any combination of radon daughters in 1 liter of air whose radioactive decay will result in the release of 130,000 million electron volts of alpha-particle energy.

Index

Index